Y0-BDO-683

AFFECTIVE EDUCATION IN NURSING

A Guide to Teaching and Assessment

Elizabeth C. King, Ph.D.

Dean, College of Health and Human Services
Eastern Michigan University
Ypsilanti, Michigan

AN ASPEN PUBLICATION ®
Aspen Systems Corporation
Rockville, Maryland
Royal Tunbridge Wells
1984

Library of Congress Cataloging in Publication Data

King, Elizabeth C., 1941–
Affective education in nursing.

An Aspen publication.
Includes index.
1. Nursing—Psychological aspects—Study and teaching.
2. Nursing—Moral and ethical aspects—Study and teaching.
3. Nursing—Psychological aspects—Case studies.
4. Nursing—Moral and ethical aspects—Case studies.
I. Title. [DNLM: 1. Education, Nursing. 2. Affect—
Nursing texts. WY 18 K508a]
RT86.K48   1984   610.73 '01 '9   83-9235
ISBN: 0-89443-888-3

Publisher: John Marozsan
Editorial Director: Darlene Como
Executive Managing Editor: Margot Raphael
Editorial Services: Scott Ballotin
Printing and Manufacturing: Debbie Collins

Library of Congress Catalog Card Number: 83-9235
ISBN: 0-89443-888-3

Printed in the United States of America

1   2   3   4   5

To my mother
Louise Camp, R.N.
and
my sister
Joanna F. Hofmann, R.N., M.S.N.

Table of Contents

Foreword ix

Preface xiii

Chapter 1—Rationale for Affective Education 1

Terminology 2
Moral Development and Education 4
Implications of the Theory 10
Criticisms of the Theory 11
Values Clarification 11
Implications of the Theory 16
Support of Values Clarification 17
Criticisms of Values Clarification 18
Values Inquiry 19
Implications of the Theory 22
Criticism of Values Inquiry 22
Normative and Applied Ethics 23
Appendix 1-A 28
Appendix 1-B 38

Chapter 2—Systematic Instructional Design 41

The Rationale Statement 43
Goals and Objectives 44
Developing Affective Objectives: A Taxonomy 48
Preassessment of Students' Learning 60
Learning Strategies 62
Media for Instructional Use 65

Postassessment of Behavioral Changes 66
Instructional Revision 67

Chapter 3—Classroom Teaching Strategies **71**

Group Discussion 71
The Case Study Method 85
Examples of Case Studies 88
Role Playing 95
Examples of Role-Playing Exercises 99
Simulation Gaming 108
Appendix 3-A 118
Appendix 3-B 125
Appendix 3-C 131

Chapter 4—Construction of Assessment Instruments **141**

Psychometric Orientation to Attitudes 142
The Likert Scale 143
The Semantic Differential Scale 148
The Thurstone Scale 156
Limitations of Attitude Measures 162
Behavioral Orientation Assessment 164
Rating Scales 164
Guidelines for Constructing Scales 169
Variables Affecting Validity, Reliability 173
Checklists: Types and Uses 176
Suggestions for Preparing Checklists 179
Checklists and Self-Assessment 181
Variables Affecting Validity, Reliability 182
Anecdotal Records 182
Advantages and Limitations of Data 183
Guidelines for Anecdotal Recording 186
Variables Affecting Validity, Reliability 188
Counseling Orientation 189
The Information-Oriented Interview 189
Information-Oriented Interview Guidelines 192
The Experiential Interview 194
Affective Skills 196
Communication Skills 198
Behavior Modification Interview 202
Suggestions for Effective Interviewing 202

Adapting Traditional Evaluation Methods 207
Supply-Type Test Items 208
Guidelines for Multiple-Choice Items 210
Essay Test Items 212
Guidelines for Writing Essay Test Items 213
Scoring Essay Test Items 214
Appendix 4-A 221
Appendix 4-B 226
Appendix 4-C 229
Appendix 4-D 236

Chapter 5—Instructional Revision 241

Program Evaluation Model 242
Techniques for Process Evaluation 244
The Student Rating Form 246
Assessing Faculty Advisory Role 251
Assessing Instructional Planning 252
Techniques for Product Evaluation 254
Using Results To Encourage Change 256
Appendix 5-A 258
Appendix 5-B 262
Appendix 5-C 267

Index 271

Foreword

Affective Education in Nursing: A Guide to Teaching and Assessment is the end of a process that evolved over more than two years. As the editor of *Nurse Educator,* I was asked by Dr. King about my interest in a nursing book on teaching and assessing affective education. At the time, I felt the nursing literature offered a limited, but rapidly expanding, amount of information related to the nature and value of humanistic, affective education. However, it was lacking in practical applications of the theoretical material.

When I asked why *Affective Education in Nursing* would be any different from, or more significant than, the existing literature, Dr. King replied that her approach would provide an in-depth exploration of two of the more difficult areas of curriculum design in the affective domain—teaching strategies and assessment methodologies.

As a former baccalaureate nursing educator, I was well aware of the difficulty of teaching in the affective domain and, more importantly, of trying to evaluate learning outcomes systematically and fairly. I also knew that cognitively understanding affective concepts was much easier than implementing them. It was (and is) far less threatening to think and do than it was to feel, especially when patient care or student-centered situations challenged long-held values and beliefs. Seeing the potential in a book that proposed to address these issues, I encouraged Dr. King to proceed.

I felt then, and still do, that the nature of nursing demands that educators and practitioners pay a great deal more attention to the affective components of teaching and learning. Just as different patients react differently to the same illness, based on their value system, so educators and students approach the nursing program with certain beliefs, attitudes, values, and expectations. Professionals are aware that the emotional climate set by two or more people influences the degree to which beliefs and values are rigidly protected (making new learning difficult) or are open to reexamination (and new learning). They also know how attitudes and beliefs affect, often unconsciously, daily behavior.

If for no other reasons than these, educators have the responsibility and obligation to bring values, attitudes, feelings, and beliefs into conscious awareness. Design of the curriculum can establish the learning climate that will facilitate students' ability to examine their feelings and emotions critically, to understand the hidden motivators of their behavior, and to make choices and decisions based on self-awareness and self-understanding. Reading Dr. King's manuscript, I was pleased to discover that it provided the specific information, tools, and strategies needed to develop the type of curriculum necessary for this affective growth and development.

As affective curriculum components are developed, another and often neglected issue arises: If educators are going to teach in the affective domain, they, too, must be open to examining their own value systems. It often is difficult for educators to permit people, especially those who are less experienced and younger, to feel differently about certain concepts such as trust, intimacy, justice, and the value of life.

How willing are educators to examine their own attitudes? How open are they to letting students discover their own meaning in experiences? How willing are they to accept people whose value system differs significantly from theirs? How much of their hidden selves are they willing to share with their students? Are educators as transparent as they expect their students to be?

To develop students effectively in the affective domain—to bring moral, value, and ethical issues to the forefront—nursing educators must be willing to be active participants in the learning/teaching process. They, too, have to readjust their thinking and be willing to give up old ways of perceiving and conceptualizing and realize that "these painful reorganizations are what is known as learning, and that though painful they always lead to a more satisfying and somewhat more accurate way of seeing life" (Carl R. Rogers. *On Becoming a Person.* Boston: Houghton Mifflin Co., 1961, p. 25).

Reading Dr. King's book with these thoughts in mind, I became aware of the diverse ways in which its content will be useful to nurse educators. It has significant value in helping to strengthen curriculum design pedagogically in the affective domain. It presents teaching strategies, evaluation techniques, self-assessment tools, and practical examples that will be useful to both experienced and inexperienced teachers. It truly is a step forward in understanding the value of affective education in nursing and in operationalizing important affective concepts.

Finally, and perhaps most importantly, the format provides the opportunity for nurse educators to examine their own attitudes, beliefs, and values about themselves, their teaching, and their profession. As they use *Affective Education in Nursing* to help their students become more sensitive caregivers, they will discover the benefit of getting to know themselves better through increasing their own ethical, value, and moral awareness.

Suzanne Smith Coletta
Editor of *Nurse Educator*
and the *Journal of Nursing Administration*

Preface

The idea for *Affective Education in Nursing: A Guide to Teaching and Assessment* began while the author was teaching nursing students preparing to become educators. Developing instructional materials for the affective domain was particularly frustrating. No book existed that combined teaching and evaluation strategies for that area. Consequently this work is designed to provide nursing instructors with strategies for preparing for classroom instruction and for evaluating it for the affective domain.

At the outset, the rationale for affective learning is discussed. The writings of Dewey, Piaget, Kohlberg, and others are analyzed to illustrate the strong interdependence among cognitive, psychomotor, and affective learning. This interdependence must be acknowledged if health care delivery is to be transformed from a mechanistic and disease-modeled approach to a humanistic philosophy that views body, mind, and spirit as inseparable.

Chapter 1 illustrates the belief that it is morally and pedagogically correct to teach about ethics and the skills of moral analysis. It stresses the development and enhancement of the conscious process of moral reasoning, not the teaching of a predetermined set of values. While there is value in studying the experts, what individuals believe is equally important. Once in touch with those beliefs, individuals can test them with associates through further practice and reading and in the clinical setting. The discussion and exercises on values clarification and values inquiry are intended to help implement these beliefs.

Chapter 2 summarizes the systematic approach to instructional design. It provides instructors with a strategy for integrating the components of effective instruction into overall curriculum planning and design.

Chapter 3 encourages instructors to venture beyond the typical lecture/ discussion format to include other teaching strategies that are especially useful for affective learning: group discussion, case studies, role playing, and simulation gaming. These strategies assist in the exploration of such concepts as dignity, cooperation, trust, acceptance, respect for individual differences, compromise, and truth. If affective objectives are to be met, instructors must go beyond the lecture. There is little question that modeling or social imitation learning is a powerful technique for humanistic education. The teaching strategies offered here provide a framework in which social imitation learning can occur.

Chapter 4 presents four orientations to affective assessment: (1) the psychometric, (2) the behavioral, (3) the counseling, and (4) the traditional approaches. It is designed to assist instructors in quantifying subjective data. Evaluating affective learning is difficult. However, the chapter offers a variety of evaluation techniques that are available and can be used successfully. To evaluate affective objectives, grading is deemphasized and the development of the student is made the primary concern.

Affective Education in Nursing ends by asking the questions, "How do educators determine whether their goals and objectives were met? If met, were they appropriate? Were the instructional methods effective? In summary, did they accomplish what they planned?" Chapter 5 is based on the philosophy that instructors can fail to meet an objective or goal yet not be failures, that they are willing to begin again and to keep and repeat what was successful and to search for new ways to overcome what was unsuccessful. While educators cannot make students become more humanistic nurses, they can provide the setting and experiences for that learning.

The author's hope for instructors using this text is that they will find suggestions for implementing the affective objectives they believe essential for humanistic nursing care so that their students graduate with both a feeling of being and a reason for being.

A few notes on content:

Unless identified otherwise, all exhibits, tables, and figures are by the author.

In Chapter 2, the opening section and the segment on "Learning Strategies" are adapted from *Classroom Evaluation Strategies* by this author, with permission from the C. V. Mosby Company, St. Louis, copyright © 1979.

In Chapter 3, the "Directed Role-Playing Exercise" involving Belinda and a CAT scanner is adapted from *Any Other Song: A Plea for Holistic Communications* by E. L. Daniel, published by the Robert J. Brady Company, Bowie, Md., copyright © 1980, with permission of the Robert J. Brady Company.

In Chapter 4, the final section, on "Adapting Traditional Evaluation Methods," is adapted from the author's article titled "Constructing Classroom Achievement Tests" in *Nurse Educator,* September–October 1978, *3,* 30–36, with permission of that journal, copyright © 1978.

In Chapter 5, material on teacher evaluation forms is adapted, with permission, from the work of Dr. Robert C. Wilson, Teaching Innovation and Evaluation Services, 339 Campbell Hall, University of California, Berkeley, Calif. 94220.

I would like to express my appreciation to those who assisted in the development of this book. Thank you: To the writers whose ideas are acknowledged in this text; to Darlene Como, editorial director of nursing texts at Aspen Systems, who saw some potential in the partially completed manuscript; to Teresa Hyatt, for typing and retyping the many manuscript revisions; and to Paul, Thomas, and John, for sharing in my pleasure while I was writing and upon completion of the book.

Elizabeth C. King

Chapter 1

Rationale for Affective Education

[The teacher] if he is indeed wise, he does not bid you enter the house of his wisdom, but rather leads you to the threshold of your own mind.

Kahlil Gibran

What we need in our society is nicer people; people who are richer on the inside than they are on the outside, people with more trust and tenderness, people who care for and share with one another, who have the capacity to discover and appreciate the worth of others and who are not disturbed by differences in background, behavior, and life styles; people who, when they knock on themselves, find someone at home whom they like; in short, people who want to be better human beings in a more humane community (Nyquist, 1976, p. 275).

Facilitating the development of ethical, moral, and value awareness in students sometimes is a controversial topic in nursing education because it deals with such fundamental concerns that the potential solutions may arouse deep disputes.

Trow (1976) argues that the practice and discipline of good scholarship itself contributes to the moral development of students. He suggests that since the scholar is required to listen with an open mind, consider other points of view, and engage in self-criticism that morality through scholarship occurs naturally. Consequently "morality of scholarship" is taught indirectly. That view does not recommend integration of ethical, moral, or value awareness with specific course content on the ground that learning based on scholarship is in itself a moral education. In contrast, critics argue that it cannot be concluded that moral values in scholarly work will guarantee students' moral development. Scholars' search for knowledge

1

specific to their discipline does not necessarily transfer to their personal conduct in relationships with patients and students.

Many nursing educators support the belief that students should be challenged to make choices, to probe, examine, and scrutinize ethical questions, and emerge with their own answers. Ideally, their answers will be the result of rigorous preparation in ethical, moral, and value awareness. This preparation will promote the formation of character as well as the development of intellect.

Educators are reexamining their curricula and there seems to be a strong consensus that they no longer can graduate students without spending time seriously examining and critically exploring ethical and value-laden concerns.

The increasing complexity of contemporary life and the emergence of new ethical dilemmas have created a renewed need for educators to begin to question themselves and to be concerned about the professional values of their students.

There are several variations in the approaches to moral education. The purpose here is to introduce a broad theoretical overview of four proposals on the theory and practice of moral and values education:

1. moral development and education
2. values clarification
3. values inquiry
4. normative and applied ethics.

TERMINOLOGY

The definition of terms in Exhibit 1-1 is suggested for educators designing curricula to include objectives in the affective domain. While these definitions make some distinctions, there also are some overlapping concepts. Educators write "affective" objectives in an effort to prepare more "humanistic" nurses. Moral values and judgments are aspects of affective behavior related to values involving human rights, welfare, and justice. For example, recurrent nursing issues that are aspects of moral values and judgments include these:

- Should medical treatment be withheld from a seriously deformed newborn?
- Should psychiatric patients be forced to take psychotropic medications?
- Should terminally ill adult patients have the right to know the seriousness of their illness?

Exhibit 1-1 Definitions in Affective Education

Affective: feeling or emotion.

Affective Behavior: conduct that reflects attitudes, values, beliefs, needs, and emotional responses (Davis, 1981).

Ethical Dilemma: a situation that arises when acting on one moral conviction (e.g., giving treatment) can mean breaking another (e.g., truthtelling).

Ethics: a branch of philosophy dealing with values related to human conduct, to the rightness and wrongness of certain actions, and to the goodness and badness of the motives and ends of such actions.

Humanistic: any system or mode of thought in which human interests, values, and dignity are taken to be of primary importance, as in moral judgments.

Morality: relationships between individuals and how they ought to behave toward one another (Purtilo & Cassel, 1981).

Moral Behavior: conduct that results from serious critical thinking about how individuals ought to treat others; moral behavior reflects the way a person interprets basic respect for other persons, such as for respect for human life, freedom, justice or confidentiality (Davis, 1981).

Moral Education: the direct and indirect intervention of the curriculum to affect moral behavior and the capacity to develop moral reasoning skills; because moral education considers fundamental human concerns, it is capable of arousing deep controversies; whatever program of moral education is adopted, it must respect the pluralistic traditions of the United States and be free of indoctrination (Purpel & Ryan, 1975).

Nonmoral Behavior: conduct that results from reflective thinking about the values individuals hold but does not relate to how they treat others; for example, personal beliefs about dress, money, or the use of time reflect nonmoral behavior (Davis, 1981).

Normative or Applied Ethics: an approach that seeks to consider and justify what ought to be done in a given moral situation by way of clarification, analysis, and critiques of moral arguments to develop the capacity for moral reasoning.

Value Behavior: conduct based on a reflective, predetermined awareness of chosen and prized values that may be moral (i.e., relating to treatment of others) or nonmoral (i.e., belief about dress, etc.).

Values Clarification: a method of self-discovery by which people identify their personal values and their value rankings.

Values Inquiry: an approach for exploring the meaning and possibilities of a human situation by finding in it the values that motivate individuals' behavior.

In contrast, nonmoral values and judgments are related more directly to personal preferences, to goals instrumental to the profession, and to aesthetics. For example, a practitioner may prefer pediatric to medical-surgical nursing or a faculty member may prefer delivering professional services rather than doing research. Identifying the category to which the behavior belongs is a start in developing appropriate affective objectives and in planning learning experiences.

MORAL DEVELOPMENT AND EDUCATION

When considering moral education, some theorists use the term "development" to describe a systematic theory of hierarchical stages of cognitive moral growth; others refer to the formation of certain human capacities, relationships, and skills. These approaches are combined by blending moral matters and education in the broad process of human growth and development (Morrill, 1980).

The writings of John Dewey (cited in Archambault, 1964) and Jean Piaget (1948) significantly influenced the theory of cognitive moral development advanced later by Kohlberg (1975). The following discussion briefly describes Dewey's and Piaget's respective three levels or stages of moral development. It also illustrates how these theories provided the conceptual framework for Kohlberg's work.

Dewey believed that the aim of education should be both intellectual and moral growth. He viewed intellectual and moral growth as progressing through sequential, cumulative, and hierarchical developmental stages. He postulated three levels of moral development:

1. Premoral or Preconventional Level: Behavior is motivated by biological and social impulses.
2. Conventional Level: An individual's behavior reflects the standard of the group; behavior is accepted with little critical reflection.
3. Autonomous Level: An individual's behavior reflects critical thinking and judging to determine what is good; the standard of the group is not accepted without reflection.

While Dewey's approach was theoretical, Piaget made the first effort to define stages of moral reasoning in children through interviewing and observing them in games with rules. Based upon his research findings, Piaget defined levels of moral development as follows:

Stage 1: Premoral Stage. No sense of obligation to rules.
Stage 2: Heteronomous Stage (approximately 4 to 8 years). Literal obedience to rules; an equation of obligation with submission to power and punishment.
Stage 3: Autonomous Stage (approximately 8 to 12 years). Purpose and consequences of following rules are considered; obligation is based upon reciprocity and exchange.

Kohlberg (1975), like Piaget, conducted interviews in which he asked his subjects to reason out hypothetical moral dilemmas. Analyzing the responses, he concluded that moral reasoning developed through a series of six stages. For 12 years Kohlberg followed the same group of boys, checking on their development at three-year intervals from early adolescence through young adulthood. Drawing upon the work of Dewey and Piaget, he produced a more complete discussion with stages of moral development. The stages are intended to be hierarchical and are presented from lowest to highest:

Preconventional
- Stage 1.0. Obedience/punishment orientation
- Stage 2.0. Personal interest orientation

Conventional
- Stage 3.0. Good boy/nice girl orientation
- Stage 4.0. Law-and-order orientation

Postconventional
- Stage 5.0. Social contract orientation
- Stage 6.0. Conscience orientation.

The following discussion describes each level of Kohlberg's moral development theory.

Preconventional

At this level children are responsive to cultural rules and labels of good/bad, right/wrong. Behavior is interpreted in terms of its consequences (i.e., punishment or reward). The primary motivation for behavior is to avoid punishment, obtain rewards, and/or have favors returned. The primary concern is self.

Stage 1.0: Obedience/Punishment Orientation

In this stage the individual's behavior is determined mainly by an unquestioning obedience to a powerful authority. Fear of punishment dominates conduct. Stage 1 individuals do not question authority. Consequently the physical effects of their actions determine whether it is good or bad, regardless of their morality. For example, Sean may not steal because he fears punishment, not because he values honesty. Stage 1 individuals may even believe it is fine to steal if they can avoid getting caught and thereby avoid punishment.

Stage 2.0: Personal Interest (or Instrumental-Relativist) Orientation

The basic motivation for many actions is to satisfy personal needs. People view human relations in terms of reciprocity; they do not consider the needs of others unless they benefit themselves. While they may be beginning to develop a sense of fairness, their concern still is primarily for self. The reciprocity is in terms of "You help me and I'll help you." Loyalty and justice are not concerns of Stage 2 behavior.

Conventional Level

At this level, maintaining the expectations of family, group, and/or nation is desirable regardless of immediate or future consequences. Attitude is conformity and loyalty. Although control of conduct is external, motivation is largely internal.

Stage 3.0: Good Boy/Nice Girl (or Interpersonal Concordance) Orientation

Stage 3 individuals are conformists. Their behavior is aimed toward pleasing others so they will gain acceptance. Even if the behavior is bungled, it is ultimately judged by intention. This stage prepares individuals for developing a social conscience.

Stage 4.0: Law-and-Order Orientation

These individuals focus on maintaining social order. They are loyal to existing laws and promote adherence to them. Their orientation is toward authority and predetermined rules. They may admit that the system has flaws but only because everyone is not loyal to those laws.

Postconventional Level

Individuals at this stage, also called the autonomous or principled level, accept the possibility of conflict between socially accepted standards and individual moral values and principles. They attempt to make moral decisions based upon inner judgments regarding right and wrong. As a result of this autonomous thinking, moral principles have validity apart from the authority of the groups and/or individuals who hold them.

Stage 5.0: Social Contract (or Legalistic) Orientation

A more completely developed moral behavior emerges at this level. Stage 5 individuals describe behavior in terms of standards that have been agreed upon by society. However, there now are no legal absolutes. The individuals may work to change the law for the sake of society. The United States Constitution is written in Stage 5 terms.

Stage 6.0: Universal-Ethical-Principle (or Conscience) Orientation

Stage 6 individuals make decisions guided by self-chosen ethical principles. What is right is a decision of their conscience based upon ideas that apply to everyone (all nations, peoples, etc.). These are called ethical principles. An ethical principle is different from a rule (i.e., Thou shall not steal); instead, it is general (i.e., All persons are created equal). Consequently, these ethical principles are not concrete moral rules like the Ten Commandments. Behavior is based upon universal principles of justice, equality, and dignity of human beings as individuals. These principles are higher than any given law because they come from the experience of all people.

The tradition of moral philosophy that is inherent in Stage 6 is similar to the writing of Immanuel Kant (1964). Kant suggests that morality is principled (i.e., judgments are made in terms of universal principles applicable to all humankind). Principles are in contrast to rules such as the Ten Commandments. For example, two of Kant's principles are as follows:

1. Respect for human personality: "Act always toward the other as an end, not as a means."
2. Maxim of universalization: "Choose only as you would be willing to have everyone choose in your situation." In other words, individuals should choose as though they did not know what their position was to be in society and in which they might be the most disadvantaged. For example, assume a patient is comatose, terminally ill, or quadriplegic. The nurse's responsibility would be to make hospital policies that would consider the needs and desires of this totally disadvantaged patient.

The best known of Kohlberg's cases, "Heinz's dilemma," serves as a way to illustrate the approach.

> *Background:* Heinz's wife is dying of a disease that might be cured by medication that a druggist is willing to sell—but at an unfair and exorbitant price. Heinz cannot afford the medicine so he steals it.

> *Question:* Should Heinz have stolen the drug?

Various responses to the question would be given at Kohlberg's levels of cognitive moral development:

Preconventional Level
> *Stage 1:* Avoidance of punishment and deference to power form the basis of moral decisions. Example: Individuals at this stage

would expect to be caught by the police and punished for theft.

Stage 2: The basic motive is to satisfy personal needs. Individuals will not consider the needs of others unless they will benefit themselves. Example: Individuals at this stage would be less concerned with external punishment but would claim taking the drug would be wrong because of the pain and discomfort to them that would result—stealing might lead to imprisonment.

Conventional Level

Stage 3: What is approved of in terms of conventional norms is the basis for moral decisions. Example: Individuals would judge Heinz to be justified in stealing if his friends and acquaintances would reward and praise him for his actions.

Stage 4: Maintaining social order becomes the basis for moral decisions. Example: Individuals at this stage would censure theft of any sort as destructive to the legal order of society.

Postconventional Level

Stage 5: This involves a more completely developed moral behavior that sees no legal absolutes and that believes changes in the law can be made. Personal values and opinions are regarded as the basis for moral decisions. Example: Individuals at this stage would separate the legal and moral requirements of the situation. The value of life would be seen as transcending the value of property. As a result, the theft would be viewed as a morally right and responsible action. However, at Stage 5 the conflict between legal and moral claims still would be acute.

Stage 6: What is right is a decision of conscience based upon ethical principles. Example: This stage is developmentally and morally superior to the preceding ones. The value of life would be seen as transcending that of property. No internal conflict between law and moral claims would be felt. This stage coincides with the moral universalism of Kant and Rawls (1971) and can be justified in terms of their theories.

A second example illustrates Kohlberg's stages of cognitive moral development with relevant nursing content.

Background: Paul K. is recovering from a stroke. No further progress can be documented; consequently, treatments and reimbursement for them from Medicare will be discontinued.

However, Nurse C. believes that Mr. K. has only reached a temporary plateau and will continue making progress if he continues to receive treatment; if treatment is discontinued, a substantial loss of functioning is likely to occur. Nurse C. falsely reports that Mr. K. is continuing to make progress.

Question: Should Nurse C. have lied on the progress report?

According to Kohlberg, various responses would be given at different levels of cognitive moral development:

Preconventional Level

Stage 1: Avoidance of punishment and deference to power form the basis of moral decisions. Example: Individuals at this stage would expect to be caught and punished for misuse of Medicare funds.

Stage 2: The basic motive is to satisfy personal needs. Individuals will not consider the needs of others unless they will benefit themselves. Example: Individuals at this stage would be less concerned with external punishment but would assert that lying on the progress report would be wrong because of the pain and discomfort to them that would result: misuse of federal funds can lead to a large fine or imprisonment.

Conventional Level

Stage 3: What is approved in terms of conventional norms is the basis for moral decisions. Example: Individuals would judge Nurse C. to be justified in lying if her professional peers would reward and praise her for her actions.

Stage 4: Maintaining social order becomes the basis for moral decisions. Example: Individuals at this stage would censure lying of any kind as destructive to the legal order of society.

Postconventional Level

Stage 5: This involves a more completely developed moral behavior that sees no legal absolutes and that believes changes in the law can be made. Personal values and opinions are regarded as the basis for moral decisions. Example: Individuals at this stage would separate the legal and moral requirements of the situation. The potential increased quality of Mr. K.'s life would be seen as transcending the value of truthtelling. As a result, the lie would be viewed as a morally right and responsible action. However, at Stage 5, the conflict between legal and moral claims still would be acute.

Stage 6: What is right is a decision of conscience based upon ethical principles. Example: This stage is developmentally and morally superior to the preceding ones. The potential increased quality of Mr. K.'s life would be seen as transcending truthtelling. No internal conflict between law and moral claims would be felt. At this stage the individual may work to change the law.

Other individuals have espoused the highest level of moral development—Gandhi, Albert Schweitzer, Martin Luther King, Pope John, and Martin Buber. While they were from different religious faiths, their ethical principles did not conflict.

IMPLICATIONS OF THE THEORY

Erickson and Weaver (1978) suggest that less than a third of all adults appear to develop postconventional forms of moral reasoning (i.e., Stages 5 and 6). Similarly, Kohlberg (1975) contends that most individuals, regardless of age, fail to advance to the highest levels of moral reasoning. The majority of adults are said to be at Stages 3 and 4 with fewer than 10 percent of them reaching Stage 5 and 6. Kohlberg says consistent Stage 6 reasoning is rare.

If these statistics were accepted, much could be accomplished in health science education to promote moral development. Educational researchers have gathered some evidence that it is possible to promote change in moral judgment through specific instructional methods (Erickson & Weaver, 1977–1978). Kohlberg has concluded that if discussions of moral dilemmas and/or case studies involve an appropriate degree of cognitive dissonance, these analyses can accelerate the movement from one stage of cognitive moral development to another. This fundamentally assumes that the right educational approach can encourage the process of moral development.

Kohlberg's theory of moral development is humanistic, placing humans at the center of the universe, encouraging free thought and scientific inquiry, and offering no absolute standards of ethics. Individuals are challenged to analyze issues based on the concept that decisions are influenced through the use of reason. Every moral law is abstract in relation to unique and totally concrete situations. The cognitive skills of moral analysis can be gained through cognitive moral education.

Cognitive moral analysis requires a thorough knowledge and understanding of the facts of ethics and some study of its nature, origin, and foundation. Crisham's (1981) nursing research findings based on Kohlberg's cognitive theory of moral development verify the relationship of formal education to enhanced principled thinking. Crisham (1981) has developed a *Nursing Dilemma Test* to measure responses to recurrent moral dilemmas. From 130 staff nurse interviews, 21 recurrent professional moral dilemmas were identified and grouped according to four underlying ethical issues: (1) determining the right to decide, (2) defining and promoting quality of life, (3) maintaining professional and institutional standards, and (4) distributing nursing resources. Crisham (1981) finds that formal moral education has an impact on nurses' ethical decision making in actual clinical practice.

CRITICISMS OF THE THEORY

Some critics suggest that it is not right to assert the superiority of Kantian ethics (i.e., Stage 6) over utilitarian views (i.e., Stage 5). They argue that philosophers have spent lifetimes studying Kantian ethics and utilitarian views and have not found the philosophical base to support a hierarchical ranking. The gap between reason and action thus still remains. Individuals can reason at Stage 6 yet still act egocentrically (Morrill, 1980).

Kohlberg's theory does not respond sufficiently to the body of research in biology, sociology, and psychology that describes how drives, pressures, conditioning, and emotional conflicts control human behavior (Lickona, 1976). Kohlberg's approach also does not involve a particular moral subject matter or discipline, such as philosophy. This limits its wide and direct application to health science education. However, the theoretical base can be used to suggest a pedagogical approach to existing subject matter.

Regardless of the criticism of Kohlberg's theory, it does provide a theoretical base that can be used in a pedagogical approach to consider moral situations. Movement to higher stages of moral development is advantageous not only to the individual but also to society.

VALUES CLARIFICATION

Values clarification is another variation in the approaches to moral education. By definition, values clarification is a method of self-discovery by which persons identify their personal values and value rankings. The basic objective is to enhance personal growth through heightened self-awareness.

Nurses deal daily, often minute by minute, with situations that require value judgments. However, some nursing educators may fail to discuss the impact of personal values and feelings on professional behavior. The revised *Code for Nurses* (1976), Item 1, states: "The nurse provides services with respect for human dignity and the uniqueness of the client unrestricted by consideration of social or economic status, personal attributes, or the nature of health problems." Students are led to believe that they will be able to provide equally to all persons in all situations.

In reality, the myth of value-free professional behavior may prevent instructors from discussing the potential impact of personal attitudes and values on the delivery of patient care. Furthermore, it prevents the discussion of alternative actions in situations demanding triage. Finally, it allows personal values to be hidden and nurses to remain oblivious to the effects of attitudes and values on the delivery of care.

Personal attitudes and values do have an impact on both patient care and curriculum planning. Since daily decisions may have life-and-death implications, consideration of how personal values influence decision making is crucial.

Raths, Harmin, and Simon (1966) provide the theoretical context of values clarification by centering on the valuing process—on the way people arrive at their values—rather than on the content of the values they choose. They stress that holding a value involves an active process of choosing and prizing beliefs and acting on them. Like Kohlberg, their writings have been influenced by Dewey.

The most influential theorists and practitioners of values clarification stress seven criteria of the valuing process (Raths, Harmin, & Simon, 1966; Simon & Kirschenbaum, 1972), as shown in Exhibit 1-2. These criteria are discussed next. By applying them, it is possible to observe and distinguish between values and other forms of human behavior. For example, if an individual professes a belief but does not act upon it, or refuses to affirm it publicly, the criteria of the valuing process have not been met.

1. *Choosing freely:* Many of the values that individuals hold were developed as the result of behavior that was done to gain approval, hold or gain love, and enhance self-esteem. These value patterns were introjected rather than evolving from within the person. As a result individuals learn to distrust their own experience as a guide to behavior. Because these learned concepts are not based upon an individual mature value system, they tend to be rigid and fixed (Rogers, 1969).

For example, some value patterns that may be introjected as desirable or undesirable are:

• Sexual desires and behaviors are mostly bad.
• Disobedience is bad.

Exhibit 1-2 Valuing Process Criteria

Choosing One's Beliefs and Behaviors

1. Choosing freely
2. Choosing from among alternatives
3. Choosing after consideration of the consequences

Prizing One's Beliefs and Behaviors

4. Prizing and cherishing
5. Affirming

Acting on One's Beliefs

6. Acting upon choices
7. Repeating

Source: Raths, L.E., Harmin, M., & Simon, S.B. *Values and Teaching.* Columbus, Ohio: The Charles E. Merrill Publishing Co., Inc., 1966. pp. 6, 170–171, 197–200.

- Making money is the highest good.
- Loving thy neighbor is the highest good.
- Cooperation and teamwork are preferable to acting alone.

When values are introjected and developed to gain approval of others:

- The majority of the individuals' values come from others but they regard them as their own.
- The source of evaluation on most matters lies outside the individual.
- The criteria by which the individuals' values are set are determined by the degree to which expression of these values will result in love and/or acceptance.
- The locus of evaluation of these patterns is external and the individuals have not developed their own valuing process, so they may feel insecure and easily threatened when their value system is questioned. Consequently, they may hold values more rigidly (Rogers, 1969).

Rogers suggests that this description of the individual with values mostly introjected, held as fixed concepts, and rarely examined or tested, is true for most persons. Before individuals can begin to develop an approach to a mature value system and not adopt the values of significant others, they must see themselves as persons who have worth. They must believe they are prized as individuals and valued for their separateness and uniqueness. When this happens they can begin to use their own feeling and experiences as a guide to determining their own behavior.

The implications of this fact are important to educators. For educators to be effective in implementing value-laden teaching/learning strategies in the classroom, they first must respect all individuals for their own uniqueness. Instructors' recognition of this prerequisite criterion will assist students in the critical thinking necessary to make value-related decisions. Values must be selected freely if they are to be truly personal.

2. *Choosing from among alternatives:* Only when a choice is possible when there is an alternative to choose from can a value result.

For example, it makes no sense to report that an individual values food, warmth, and shelter for these are basic human needs. What may be valued is a certain type of food, or a certain type of shelter, but not eating and shelter themselves. People must have food and shelter to exist; only when there is an alternative can a value result.

3. *Choosing after consideration of the consequences:* For the mature individual the moment of experiencing contains hypotheses about the consequences (Rogers, 1969). "I would enjoy sleeping with you but how would I feel about it tomorrow?" Past, present, and future all are elements that are considered when making a value-laden decision.

The process of valuing is complex, the choices are difficult, and there is no guarantee that the option selected will result in a more complete, more fully developed person. However, if the chosen action is not self-enhancing it can be done differently the next time. Through discussion, the instructor can ask questions regarding the consequences of an action without criticizing the action:

- "What did you like about what you did?" This question encourages the students to take the responsibility for their actions.
- "If you could do it again, what would you do differently?" This question points out that the students can change their behavior.
- "Do you need any help from me?" This question informs the students that positive, supportive assistance is available if needed.

It should be noted that these questions eliminate any need for external criticism.

4. *Prizing and cherishing:* When value-laden decisions are prized, they tend to contribute to the individual's inner happiness. People prize and cherish their values.

5. *Affirming:* When people have chosen freely from among alternatives and after consideration of the consequences, and prize or cherish that choice, they are likely to affirm their values publicly.

6. *Acting upon choices:* For a value to be present there must be some overt behavior that demonstrates that value.

For example, if individuals are to value sincerity, they must act unpretentiously. If they value independence, they must not view pleasing others as a goal in itself. Individuals who say one thing and do another do not yet have a mature value pattern.

7. *Repeating:* Mature, developed value systems lead to patterns of behavior that are consistent in several different situations and over time.

For example, if instructors value each student as a unique individual they will treat every one with respect no matter what the situation. Values that have been internalized will appear and reappear forming fairly predictable patterns.

Values can be defined as standards of choice; they help guide individuals and groups toward meaningful lives (Morrill, 1980). As standards of choice, values are not specific things, beliefs, actions, or value judgments such as an original work of art, a belief in tolerance, a considerate action, or a decision to fail a student caught cheating. These specifics are indicators or expressions of values. However, in isolation they are not values but help form a larger construct of value-oriented choice.

Valuing is an orientation assumed by the self through prizing, choosing, and acting, all in an intricate, interrelated sequence of events. Values never are fully actualized unless they orient choice and determine behavior. Since values do in fact orient behavior, they exercise authority over individuals by demanding consistent conduct (Morrill, 1980). A purported value that fails to produce consistent action is not a value; perhaps a belief, an attitude, an ideal, but not a deeply held value. To be held as a value there must be deep personal commitment that becomes central to the individuals' identity.

IMPLICATIONS OF THE THEORY

Won't this emphasis on individuals' determining their own values create a society of conflicting values? A value, to merit the term, requires conduct that has worth, that results in the fulfillment of human potential (Morrill, 1980).

Rogers (1969) reports that in his experience in therapy, when individuals are highly valued, certain value orientations seem to emerge. These value patterns are not dependent upon the personality of the therapist nor the influences of the culture. As Rogers's clients moved in the direction of personal growth and maturity they demonstrated the following value patterns:

1. Pretense and defensiveness were valued negatively.
2. Meeting the expectations of others as a goal in itself was valued negatively.
3. Being themselves was valued highly.
4. Self-direction and choosing freely were valued highly.
5. Their self and feelings were valued highly.
6. They were sensitive to their own inner feelings and those of others; openness was valued highly.
7. Appreciation, sensitivity, and acceptance of others were valued positively.
8. Close, intimate relationships with another person were valued highly.

Rogers concludes that when individuals are prized as persons, the values that they select tend to be experiences that contribute to the growth and development of themselves and of others. Rogers believes that a culture in which individuals are highly prized also will have persons who prize and value themselves and each other. Finally, he holds that a "universality of values" can be determined not by religion, science, or philosophy but from within humans themselves. To many, this may seem to be a heretical belief; to others, it may be known already.

"Man has within himself an organismic basis for valuing. To the extent that he can be freely in touch with this valuing process in himself, he will behave in ways which are self-enhancing" (Rogers, 1969, p. 256).

As a result of today's pluralistic society, personal and professional values may conflict. The revised Code for Nurses (1976) provides guidance in delivering nursing care while at the same time respecting personal values. The code states that the nurse can refuse to participate in the delivery of care if personally opposed. However, the nurse must provide advance notice of the refusal so that alternative arrangements can be made.

In an emergency, the professional code requires that regardless of personal values, the nurse must provide the best possible care. Consequently, the professional code assumes priority over a personally held value.

SUPPORT OF VALUES CLARIFICATION

Values clarification strategies can promote affective growth as well as freedom and structure in the classroom (Costa, 1977). Freedom in the classroom in the most humanistic sense means freedom from ridicule, freedom to experiment and take personal risks in a supportive environment, and freedom to explore personal meaning.

Structure may be interpreted to mean fair ground rules, fair constraints, and honest, open communication. The more students can decide for themselves, the more humanistic the classroom. Students and instructor can structure the classroom together, deciding upon tasks to be accomplished and mutually agreeing on ground rules.

Values clarification strategies teach individuals to think through issues and to develop a personal value system through an affective and cognitive process. However, before values clarification strategies are planned for the classroom, the instructor should be certain that each student has adequate knowledge and understanding of the facts. This understanding should include a thorough examination of all sides of the issue. It is easy to underestimate the amount of information needed to analyze a moral issue competently (Scriven, 1975). For example, before discussing the issue of renal dialysis, the students should have a knowledge of normal and abnormal kidney function and its relationship to the entire body.

Instructors can learn to use values clarification teaching methods with relative ease (Kirschenbaum, 1977). There are a variety of materials available that can be adopted to all levels of education and for almost every type of student or adult. However, for instructors to benefit from a training period in value clarification methods:

- They must believe students should make their own decisions and think for themselves.
- They must refrain from assuming an authoritative role and adopt a more facilitative and listening posture.
- They must accept diversity of race, sex, values, etc., among their students. One of the greatest contributions of value clarification strategies in education has been its confrontation with traditional/authoritarian education (Stewart, 1975).

- They must be willing to accept all viewpoints unconditionally and not impose their personal values upon the students. The ability to entertain alternatives and to negotiate no-lose solutions to problems often leads to group decisions that are more beneficial for both the individual and the group.

However, while it is morally and pedagogically correct to teach about ethics and the skills of moral analysis rather than doctrine, it is not correct to imply that all the various incompatible views about such issues as abortion or nuclear power or war are equally right or deserving of respect (Scriven, 1975).

While pluralism requires respecting the rights of others to hold divergent beliefs, it does not imply tolerance of actions based upon those beliefs nor does it mean respecting the content of the beliefs. For example, some actions are morally indefensible (e.g., the Rev. Jim Jones led 911 of his People's Temple followers to their death in a mass suicide) even when done "in conscience"—that is, dictated by personal beliefs.

Many decisions are influenced implicitly or explicitly by values. Students enter postsecondary education with many attitudes and values formed during childhood. However, those late adolescent concepts generally are reshaped by the college experience. Since value formation is a lifelong process, schools have a responsibility to promote the development of affective moral education (Scott, 1978).

CRITICISMS OF VALUES CLARIFICATION

Many values clarification exercises elicit rather unimportant opinions, feelings, and personal anxieties without requiring the students to discover value patterns (Morrill, 1980). Many educators interpret values clarification primarily as a technique deficient in academic content, to be used in such areas as career planning and counseling but not important enough to integrate into the academic curriculum.

An irony inherent in the neutral, content-free position of values clarification is that it assumes self-affirmation, autonomy, trust, free choice, and tolerance as basic values. Values clarification also does not have a sufficient theoretical base to defend its own assumptions. Its emphasis on "free choice" is viewed by critics as a sure criterion for relativism (which holds that the basis of judgment is relative, differing according to events, persons, etc.).

In summary, when both the support for and criticism of values clarification are considered, it can be described as serving as a pedagogical technique to clarify the personal meaning of choices and issues. It can serve as a method for encouraging and yielding self-knowledge. Since nursing is a profession that revolves around the individual, what we value and how these values are integrated into our professional lives influence the quality of care we give (Coletta, 1978). This can hardly be criticized as an educational goal. Some sample values clarification exercises are presented in Appendix 1-A.

VALUES INQUIRY

Values inquiry is another variation in the approaches to moral education. Values inquiry involves a broad and basic form of study traditionally used in higher education. By definition, values inquiry is a method that seeks to explore the meaning and possibilities of a human situation by discovering in it the values that motivate human choice. In contrast to values clarification, which promotes the identification and clarification of personal values, values inquiry focuses on the concept of values in social and moral issues.

McGrath (1974) cites the critical need for values inquiry because today's specialized disciplines with their ever narrower discipline-specific curricula merely produce facts that are of no consequence in the lives of ordinary human beings. The loss of a broad liberal and/or general education has created a need for a specific plan for values inquiry education. This is based upon the assumption that people orient and justify their choices through a set of values. Consequently there is a need to describe, reveal, and assess values to study the human experience.

Values inquiry is a cognitive approach to moral development using issue-laden situations to explore values. The values inquiry method is a step toward a rational approach to moral education. The method elicits the students' own judgments or opinions regarding issues or situations that are value laden or in which values conflict. Values inquiry opposes indoctrination and stresses open, or Socratic, peer discussion. It also seeks to diagnose ethical dilemmas.

However, while McGrath (1974) supports the concept of open Socratic discussion, he suggests that there is a normative dimension to the choice among values. According to this view, what makes an act right is a certain fact about its results or consequences.

Case studies and value-laden incidents can provide the content for values inquiry. They also can help identify the consequences of various decisions. For example, Fraenkel (1977) recommends that after a value-laden incident has been encountered, the instructor should ask the students to respond to a predetermined sequence of questions. A value-laden incident taken from *The Herald-Leader* in Lexington, Ky., January 6, 1980 (Exhibit 1-3) illustrates the method.

Fraenkel (1977) recommends that the instructor should ask several questions in a predetermined sequence:

1. determine the facts
2. explore inferences about why the facts occurred
3. explore inferences about the individuals' value system
4. gather evidence to support the inferences.

Another approach to value inquiry focuses on a more traditional problem-solving methodology as illustrated in Exhibit 1-4.

Exhibit 1-3 Example of a Values Inquiry Incident

PARENTS BLAME THEMSELVES, THEIR RELIGION FOR SON'S DEATH

DETROIT—It has been more than two years now. And still, Doug and Rita Swan are living through "that awful nightmare."

They are not just living through it, though. They are consumed by it. Consumed by guilt, and consumed by the tragedy of a faith shattered and a young child's death.

Two years ago, in the spring of 1977, the Swans were the quintessential happy young family. At least outwardly.

Doug Swan taught math at the Detroit Institute of Technology. Rita Swan was a part-time English instructor at Wayne State University and Wayne County Community College. They lived in suburban Grosse Pointe Park. They had two children, 8-year-old Cathy and 16-month-old Matthew.

And they had religion—Christian Science—a religion they had both known and practiced since childhood. On Sundays they taught Sunday school.

When a young child dies, not even a parent who teaches Sunday school is prepared. Any typical, loving parent is crushed.

And that is what happened when Matthew Swan, age 16 months, died of spinal meningitis at 1 a.m., July 7, 1977. Rita and Doug Swan were shattered. The difference is that they blamed themselves and their religion for their son's death. And they have refused to grieve quietly.

For 12 days, fevered and lying in a near coma much of the time, Matthew Swan was kept at home after he fell ill on Father's Day weekend, June 1977.

Following their Christian Science beliefs, the Swans did not seek medical help. Prayer, faith and knowledge were to heal Matthew. A Christian Science practitioner—a person sanctioned by the church to assist in healing through prayer—was called. Prayers were offered. Matthew remained ill.

Finally, torn by fear and doubt, and realizing they were rejecting a faith long held dear, the Swans rushed their dying son to the hospital. It was too late.

Despite emergency surgery and the life-prolonging use of a respirator, Matthew Swan died within a week.

Exhibit 1-3 continued

And now Rita and Doug Swan are haunted. And angry. And still filled with anguish. They are certain their son could have been saved.

"I will always feel that guilt," Rita Swan said. "Matthew's death was not right. He was a beautiful child. He had infinite potential. It was a massive injustice that happened to him, and secondarily to us."

The Swans have spent two years working through their guilt, their massive anger. Even after a move last year to Jamestown, N.D., where she and her husband are instructors at Jamestown College, Rita Swan continues to write and rewrite a painfully emotional, 50-page account of Matthew's final days.

In December, the Swans exhibited those painful emotions and their concern about children's rights and the Christian Science church on the "Phil Donahue Show." And they have a Detroit lawyer researching the possibilities for state legislation to protect the rights of a child caught in what one person called "a religious Catch-22."

A child's death is tragic. But the issues involved here—medical, legal, religious, moral—are far more complex.

Rita and Doug Swan, native Kansans, were raised in the Christian Science church.

"We were both very involved in the church," said Doug Swan. "We were Sunday school teachers, we were officers, we wrote religious articles. We had relied on Christian Science exclusively as a means of healing. If you believe in a religion, you follow it."

The Swans carried no medical insurance.

"Christian Science," said Rita Swan, analyzing her past, "was wrapped up with my security, my marriage, my family, my happiness."

Source: Reprinted with permission from *The Herald-Leader,* Lexington, Ky., January 6, 1980.

Exhibit 1-4 Example of a Value Incident

CHILDLESS COUPLE: Wife unable to conceive, looking for woman who would agree to be artificially inseminated with semen of husband and give child to couple. All responses confidential, all expenses paid. Please state fee expected. Kindly direct responses to . . . [*The Herald-Leader,* Lexington, Ky., December 9, 1979]

Statement of the Problem: What is the problem?

Alternatives: What other alternatives did the childless couple have as options?

Consequences: What are the possible consequences of each alternative, including the chosen option?

Evidence: What evidence is there that these consequences might occur? (Note: To answer this question adequately, the students will have to do some literature review on such topics as adoption, foster care, and genetics.)

Assessment: What are the advantages and disadvantages of each consequence? Why?

Decision: What would you do if you were the "childless couple?" Why?

Source: Adapted from *How to Teach About Values* by J.R. Fraenkel, published by Prentice-Hall, Inc., Englewood Cliffs, N.J. Copyright © 1977, by permission of Prentice-Hall, Inc.

The steps used in discussing the childless couple value incident were adapted from those suggested by Fraenkel (1977) for analyzing a value dilemma.

IMPLICATIONS OF THE THEORY

By using values inquiry as a method to explore the values that motivate human choice, a new dimension of understanding others is possible. For example, a review of the literature confirms that many nurses have negative attitudes toward alcoholics (Cornish & Miller, 1976; Ferneau & Morton, 1968; Schmid & Schmid, 1973). Such findings are discouraging when it is considered that the nurses' attitudes affect their relationship with patients and the degree to which they view their practice as successful (Williams, 1979). These findings also are depressing in view of the philosophy of holistic nursing care.

However, by applying values inquiry methods, a better understanding of alcoholic patients is possible. Estes and Madden (1975) suggest the use of popular literature to illustrate the effects of alcoholism on such patients. They designed a course around the following books, all of which involve alcoholism in varying degree: *Long Day's Journey Into Night* by Eugene O'Neill, *The Razor's Edge* by Somerset Maugham, *The Lost Weekend* by Charles Jackson, and *I'll Cry Tomorrow* by Lillian Roth.

A values inquiry approach to the study of alcoholism can aid in the development of empathy, help decrease negative attitudes, and, more importantly, motivate nurses to work toward rehabilitation of such patients.

CRITICISM OF VALUES INQUIRY

It is difficult to document the claim that a full exploration of values will diminish the gap between reason and action. Values inquiry needs to develop specific criteria for assessing the analysis of values as an intellectual task. It also needs to describe the extent to which a full and clear analysis can or will affect the development of students' personal values. For example, does a full exploration of values produce a commitment to personally held values?

Regardless of the criticism, value inquiry methods can strengthen students' in-depth understanding of selected subject matter. The process requires students to gather data, consider alternatives and consequences, and increase their communication skills. Three additional values inquiry exercises are presented in Appendix 1-B.

NORMATIVE AND APPLIED ETHICS

The contemporary study of ethics traditionally has been concerned with the history or justification of ethical discussions. The discussions usually are not concerned with the specific acts of individuals but rather with the meaning of such basic ethical terms as good, right, bad, honest, etc. As a result, ethics was regarded as a rather narrow subject that did not offer much help in coping with the increasing complexity of contemporary moral questions such as the ability to detect defective fetuses in utero, the development of recombinant DNA techniques, and the use of artificial means to sustain life.

However, since the early 1970s there has been a trend toward the growth of normative ethics. In contrast to traditional ethics, normative ethics seeks to consider and justify what ought to be done in a given moral situation. Through clarification, analysis, and critiques of moral arguments, normative ethics seeks to develop students' capacities for moral reasoning. Through the study of normative and applied ethics students can increase their moral awareness and further the development of their moral identity. To help meet these objectives Bok (1976) recommends interdisciplinary courses focusing on a specific contemporary moral issue using classroom discussion as the primary teaching methodology.

Contemporary ethical theories include several different philosophical frameworks:

- Utilitarianism: This involves the ethical doctrine that virtue is based on utility and that conduct should be directed toward promoting the greatest happiness for the greatest number of people.
- Kantian Ethics: This involves the ethical doctrine that individuals should act in such a way that they always treat humanity, whether in their own person or in the person of any other, never simply as a means but at the same time as an end (Kant, 1964, p. 96). Individuals always should act toward others as an end, not as a means. Under the maxim of universalization, individuals should act as if the substance of action were to become, through their will, a universal law of nature (Kant, 1964, p. 91).
- Meta Ethics: This involves a type of moral inquiry in which individuals attempt to discover and explain the meanings of the crucial terms of moral appraisal: "good," "bad," "right," "wrong," and "obligatory."

From this it is easy to conclude that there is no consensus concerning which ethical theories to teach; however, there is agreement on both the content and the methodology.

When considering content, most ethicists conclude that the broad principles that safeguard life, property, contracts, and truthtelling should be taught. Most also agree that rational and analytical skills should be involved in moral reasoning. This analytical approach ensures critical thinking and opposes indoctrination.

Professional ethics is another area to be taught. Nursing educators have considered the impact of professional training on professional responsibility. Professional ethics has considered several types of issues: Should a nurse tell a half-truth to a patient? Disobey a superior's orders? Protect sources? Make public confidential information?

Two norms often must be reconciled in codes of professional responsibility—those of the profession itself, and general ethical principles. At one extreme are the norms of the profession equivalent to a formal etiquette of professional identity and belonging. For example, ethics in a descriptive sense describes the norms by which the group members define themselves. Even groups such as the Mafia have a set of norms; the ultimate penalty for violating them is removal from the group. At the other extreme, the professional code must encompass universal ethical principles of justice, respect for life, truthfulness, etc. (i.e., principles that apply to all persons).

In contrast to cognitive moral development, values clarification, and values inquiry, ethics is a specific field of study with characteristic forms of reasoning. However, mastery of ethics does not ensure moral actions. The study of ethics will help identify the right choice but cannot guarantee it. Furthermore, the teaching of ethics as a discipline requires a trained professional.

In summary, there is a strong interdependence between intellect and conscience, between knowledge and responsibility, that must be acknowledged to understand the nature of values (Morrill, 1980). It also must be acknowledged if educators and nurses are going to be open to reexamine their values and beliefs concerning patient care. They must transform health care delivery from a disease-modeled approach to a holistic philosophy that views body, mind, and spirit as inseparable. They need to build interdependent relationships with clearly understood individual responsibilities.

Four variations in approaches to moral education discussed were moral education and development, values clarification, values inquiry, and normative and applied ethics.

Moral education and development has been influenced by the writings of Dewey (cited in Archambault, 1964), Piaget (1948), and Kohlberg (1975). Dewey postulated three levels of moral development: (1) premoral or preconventional, (2) conventional, and (3) autonomous. Piaget proposed three stages of moral reasoning: (1) premoral, (2) heteronomous, and (3)

Table 1-1 Comparison of Cognitive Moral Development Theories

Dewey	Piaget	Kohlberg
1. *Premoral or Preconventional Level:* Behavior motivated by biological and social impulses.	*Stage 1. Premoral Stage:* No sense of obligation to rules.	*Preconventional:* Stage 1.0. Obedience/punishment orientation; Stage 2.0. Personal interest orientation.
2. *Conventional Level:* Behavior reflection of groups' standards.	*Stage 2. Heteronomous Stage:* Literal obedience to rules.	*Conventional:* Stage 3.0. Good boy/nice girl orientation; Stage 4.0. Law-and-order orientation.
3. *Autonomous Level:* Behavior independent, reflecting critical thinking.	*Stage 3. Autonomous Stage:* Purpose and consequences of rules considered.	*Postconventional:* Stage 5.0. Social contract orientation; Stage 6.0. Conscience orientation.

autonomous. Kohlberg, drawing on the work of Dewey and Piaget, identified three levels of cognitive moral development, with two stages within each level. Table 1-1 briefly compares the Dewey, Piaget, and Kohlberg cognitive moral development theories.

Values clarification is a method of self-discovery by which individuals identify their personal values and value rankings. Raths, Harmin, and Simon (1966) and Simon and Kirschenbaum (1972) have been influential theorists and practitioners of values clarification strategies. The process of valuing is complex, for if individuals are to hold a value, they must prize, choose, and act all in an intricate interrelated sequence of events. To hold a construct as a value there must be deep personal commitment that becomes central to an individual's identity.

Values inquiry is another approach to moral education. This method seeks to explore the meaning and possibilities of a human situation by discovering in it the values that motivate choice. It is a cognitive approach to moral development using value-laden situations to explore values within social and moral issues.

Normative and applied ethics also is an approach to moral education. Contemporary ethical theories include utilitarianism, Kantian ethics, many versions of religious ethics, and professional ethics. Each of these theories provides suggestions for integrating moral and values education into the nursing curriculum.

REFERENCES

American Nurses' Association. *Code for nurses with interpretive statements.* Kansas City, Mo., 1976.

Archambault, R.D. (Ed.). *John Dewey on education: Selected writings.* New York: Random House Publishing Co., Inc., 1964.

Bok, D. Can ethics be taught? *Change,* October 1976, *8,* 26–30.

Coletta, S.S. Values clarification in nursing: Why? *American Journal of Nursing,* 1978, *78*(12), 2057.

Cornish, R.D., & Miller, M.V. Attitudes of registered nurses toward the alcoholic. *Journal of Psychiatric Nursing,* December 1976, *14,* 19–22.

Costa, A.L. Affective education: The state of the art. *Educational Leadership,* 1977, *34*(4), 260–263.

Crisham, P. Measuring moral judgment in nursing dilemmas. *Nursing Research,* March–April 1981, *30*(2), 104–110.

Davis, C.M. Affective education for the health professions. *Physical Therapy,* 1981, *61*(11), 1587–1593.

Erickson, V.L., & Weaver, G.C. Implications and applications of Kohlberg's theory of moral development in today's schools. *Educational Horizons,* Winter 1977–1978, *56*(2), 60–65.

Estes, N.J., & Madden, L.P. Alcoholism in fiction: Learning from the literature. *Nursing Outlook,* August 1975, *23*(8), 517–520.

Ferneau, E.W., Jr., & Morton, E.L. Nursing personnel and alcoholism. *Nursing Research,* March–April 1968, *17,* 174–177.

Fraenkel, J.R. *How to teach about values.* Englewood Cliffs, N.J.: Prentice-Hall, Inc., 1977.

Kant, I. *Groundwork of the metaphysic of morals* (H.J. Paton, trans. and anal.). New York: Harper and Row Publishers, Inc., 1964.

Kirschenbaum, H. In support of values clarification. *Social Education,* 1977, *41*(5), 398–402.

Kohlberg, L. The cognitive-developmental approach to moral education. *Phi Delta Kappan,* June 1975, *56*(10), 670–677.

Lickona, T. (Ed.). *Moral development and behavior: Theory, research and social issues.* New York: Holt, Rinehart & Winston, Inc., 1976.

McGrath, E.J. Careers, values and general education. *Liberal Education,* 1974, *60,* 1–23.

Morrill, R.L. *Teaching values in college.* San Francisco: Jossey-Bass, Inc., Publishers, 1980.

Nyquist, E.B. The American "no fault" morality. *Phi Delta Kappan,* November 1976, *58*(3), 272–276.

Piaget, J. *The moral judgment of the child* (2nd ed.). Glencoe, Ill.: The Free Press, 1948.

Purpel, D., & Ryan, K. Moral education: Where sages fear to tread. *Phi Delta Kappan,* June 1975, *56*(10), 659–662.

Purtilo, R.B., & Cassel, C.K. *Ethical dimensions in the health professions.* Philadelphia: W.B. Saunders Company, 1981.

Raths, L.E.; Harmin, M.; & Simon, S.B. *Values and teaching.* Columbus, Ohio: The Charles E. Merrill Publishing Co., Inc., 1966.

Rawls, J. *A theory of justice.* Cambridge, Mass.: Harvard University Press, 1971.

Rogers, C.R. *Freedom to learn.* Columbus, Ohio: The Charles E. Merrill Publishing Co., Inc., 1969.

Schmid, N.J., & Schmid, D.T. Nursing students' attitudes toward alcoholics. *Nursing Research,* May–June 1973, *22*(3), 246–248.

Scott, L.J. Asking values questions in a large university: A case study. *Counseling and Values,* 1978, *22*(4), 221–237.

Scriven, M. Cognitive moral education. *Phi Delta Kappan,* June 1975, *56*(10), 689–694.

Simon, S.B., & Kirschenbaum, H. *Values clarification: A handbook of practical strategies for teachers and students.* New York: Hart Publishing Company, Inc., 1972.

Stewart, J.S. Clarifying values clarification: A critique. *Phi Delta Kappan,* June 1975, *56*(10), 684–688.

Trow, M. Higher education and moral development. *AAUP Bulletin,* 1976, *62*, 20–27.

Williams, A. The student and the alcoholic patient. *Nursing Outlook,* July 1979, *27*(7), 470–472.

Appendix 1-A

Sample Values Clarification Exercises

Regardless of how objective criteria seem to be, decisions almost always are influenced by personally held values. For example, decisions concerning admissions to a nursing program, selection of a chairman, or simply buying a car consider such criteria as valuing standardized test scores vs. autobiographical data, clinical experience vs. publication record, and comfort vs. economy. There are few decisions that are not affected by value judgments. Decision making thus is likely to be improved when the values surrounding the choice and the alternatives are explored.

Values Continuum

Directions:
Circle the number on each continuum that best applies to you.

1. How do you feel about what you wear?

1	2	3	4	5
Wrinkled Wilma or William, even when my clothes are new				Neat Nina or Norman, even iron my underwear

Sources: Values Continuum, Personal Coat of Arms, Unfinished Sentences as Value Whips, Forced-Choice Rank Ordering, and *Values Voting* adapted from *Values Clarification: A Handbook of Practical Strategies for Teachers and Students* by Sidney B. Simon, Leland W. Howe, and Howard Kirschenbaum, published by A. & W. Publishers, Inc., New York, N.Y. Copyright © 1972, by permission of Hart Publishing Company, Inc. The authors acknowledge Sr. Louise, principal of St. Julian's School, Chicago.

Values Clarification Exercises 1 and 2 adapted from classroom exercises developed by Christine Rhoda.

In *Values Clarification, Exercise 3,* the *Code for Nurses* is reprinted from *Code for Nurses with Interpretive Statements* with permission of the American Nurses' Association, Inc., © 1976.

2. How do you feel about belonging to a professional organization?

1	2	3	4	5
Loner Linda or Louis, refuse to become a member				Joiner Jane or Jim, will join as soon as possible

3. How do you feel about school?

1	2	3	4	5
Dynamite Diane or Don, students would be better off if the school were blown to bits				Scholarly Susan or Sam, loves school, has to be driven out at the end of class

4. How much do you communicate with patients?

1	2	3	4	5
Tight lipped Louise or Lincoln				Chatty Cathy or Chuck

5. What percentage of the time are you happy?

1	2	3	4	5
Sad Sara or Stan, 0 percent				Happy Helen or Harry, 100 percent

6. How clean do you keep your room?

1	2	3	4	5
Garbage dump Greta or George				Sterile Sally or Sol

7. How do you feel about conflict?

1	2	3	4	5
Shy Sara or Steve, takes off at the first sign of any trouble				Bruised Belinda or Bruce, just look at the person crosswise and you have a conflict

8. How do you handle money?

1	2	3	4	5
Tightwad Tina or Tom				Handout Hortense or Herman

9. How much do you try to please?

1	2	3	4	5
Rebel Rachael or Robert				Pleaser Pauline or Paul

This activity should be fun yet it elicits some clarification of a personal value system. Students are very creative and can create their own values continuum items.

Personal Coat of Arms

Directions:
The instructor gives each student a blank coat of arms as in the following example:

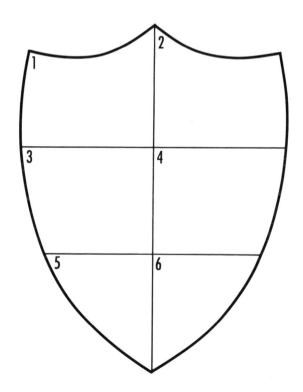

The students are asked to answer each of the following questions by drawing in the appropriate area a picture, design, or symbol that represents their response:

1. In space 1 of your coat of arms, draw three things you like to do.
2. In space 2, draw a place you go when you feel down or blue. This can be a place from your childhood that you can return to mentally or an actual place in your current environment.
3. In space 3, draw a picture, design, or symbol that represents your greatest personal achievement.
4. In space 4, draw your three biggest problems at the moment. Draw your biggest problem first, your smallest problem last.
5. In space 5, assume you have one year to live. During this year you will not be in much pain or physically handicapped. Draw what you will be doing during the coming year.
6. In space 6, assume your year to live is over. Write three adjectives that describe how you would like to be remembered. Now, write the one adjective that you would hate to have used to describe you.

To assist students in interpreting their coat of arms the instructor offers the following thoughts:

Look at space 1 and space 2 when you are having a particularly difficult time, plan some time to do the things you enjoy, and/or go to the place that offers comfort. If you cannot go there physically, do so mentally.

Look at space 4 and consider the following: your most difficult problem probably is not solvable, your second most difficult problem probably can be resolved in three to six months, and your least difficult problem probably is solvable immediately. These guidelines are generally but not always true.

Look at space 6 and enjoy the companionship of a close friend, spouse, or loved one who can be described using these adjectives. Avoid anyone who exhibits the behavior that you find unacceptable.

The instructor also can ask the students to take a close look at each response and ask themselves: What have you discovered about yourself? Were any of the questions especially difficult to answer? What values are reflected in your responses?

When using this exercise, the author assures all students at the outset that all their responses to the questions are confidential. During the discussion that follows the exercise, students are free to share or not to share their responses, as they choose.

Values Grid

Directions:

General issues are written in the left-hand column of the grid [a partial grid is below]. Next to each general issue briefly write your stand on that issue. The following seven questions are identified by number on the values grid:

1. Have you chosen your position freely?
2. Have you chosen your position after consideration of the alternatives?
3. Have you chosen your position after consideration of the consequences?
4. Are you proud of your position?
5. Have you disclosed your position to others?
6. Have you acted on your belief?
7. Have you acted repeatedly on your belief?

Place an X in the appropriate space if your answer to the question is YES.

Place an O in the appropriate space if your answer to the question is NO.

Following is a sampling of the grid:

Issue	Personal belief	1	2	3	4	5	6	7
1. Abortion (for example)	Prochoice	X	X	X	X	O	O	O
2. Confidentiality								
3. Patient rights								
4. Passive enthusiasm								
5. Etc.								

Unfinished Sentences As Value Indicators

This activity encourages students to share their feelings about a given topic. It can be used during seminars to complement clinical education experiences.

Directions:

1. Have each student complete a partially written sentence prepared by the instructor.
2. Move around the room from student to student fairly rapidly.
3. Students have the right to pass.

Possible unfinished sentences as value indicators:

1. During my clinical experience, the thing that disturbed me most was . . .
2. During my clinical experience, the thing that pleased me most was . . .
3. During clinical practice this week I wish I had . . .
4. Next week I am going to . . .

As the unfinished sentence moves from person to person around the room, everyone has the opportunity to participate or pass. It is essential that students be aware that they can pass. As they examine their own experiences and articulate their feelings, there is a growing awareness of both the commonality and variety of experiences. An unfinished sentence is a good way to start or end a class. It has the potential for involving everyone.

Forced-Choice Rank Ordering

This exercise requires students to choose from among alternatives, state or affirm their choice, and explain their position—all parts of the valuing process.

Directions:
Rank order the alternatives as follows:
   1 = first choice
   2 = second choice
   3 = third choice
Take your time. There is no *correct* ranking. Ask yourself why you believe the way you do.
Write the value that emerges in response to your *first* choice on the space as indicated.
1. Which type of patient is the most difficult for you to care for?
   _____ cancer patient
   _____ stroke patient
   _____ mentally ill patient
   _____ value(s) inherent in first choice
2. What would be the most difficult for you?
   _____ Counsel a dying child (5 to 12 years)
   _____ Counsel a dying adult (65 or older)
   _____ Counsel a parent whose child had committed suicide
   _____ value(s) inherent in first choice

3. What is the most important in a friendship?
_____ loyalty
_____ generosity
_____ honesty
_____ value(s) inherent in first choice
4. As a parent of a 15-year-old girl what would distress you most?
_____ promiscuity
_____ possession of marijuana
_____ engagement to a boy of another race
_____ value(s) inherent in first choice

Again, once the students get the idea, they will come up with forced-choice rank orderings of their own. The instructor should encourage their suggestions and use them. Each student can be asked to write one forced-choice ranking item. This will provide additional material for classroom use that is relevant to the concerns of all students.

Modification of a rank-order activity may involve assuming another role (i.e., a patient, a member of the patient's family, or a parent) before rank ordering the statements.

Values Voting

Values voting considers two steps in the valuing process: Is the individual proud and happy with the chosen value? Is the individual willing to affirm the choice publicly?
Directions:

1. If you agree, wave your hand.
2. If you disagree, place your head on the desk.
3. If you are undecided, have no feelings, or wish to pass, fold your arms across your chest.
4. The instructor then asks a series of questions or reads a series of statements. There should be no attempt to tally the responses.
5. At the end of the "voting" there should be time for students to explore areas of agreement and disagreement with each other.

Possible statements:

I would shave my beard or change my hairstyle to get a job.
I would adopt a child.
I would carry a sign in a protest march against (or for) abortion.
I would try (or refuse to try) marijuana.
I believe patients have the right to participate in all decisions related to their health care.

Once the students get the idea, they will come up with relevant statements or questions of their own. The instructor should encourage their suggestions and use them. However, it must be remembered that everyone has the right not to participate.

Values Clarification Exercise—1

You have applied for a staff nursing position at a small community long-term care nursing home. The nursing supervisor seems like a kind woman during your interview. She gives you a brief tour of the home. As you walk around, you notice many of the patients are not covered modestly. You hear one of the nurses say, "Double the valium for Mrs. Stillman, she has been noisy and demanding all day. I have lost all patience!"

The long-term nursing care facility is very close to your home, the hours are good, and the salary is competitive—but you have reservations.

What conflicting needs/values are present?

Would you accept the position?

What values would most influence your decision?

Values Clarification Exercise—2

You are the head nurse working a 4 p.m.-to-12 midnight shift in the emergency room. Following is a short profile of each patient waiting for care:

Mr. Agnew: elderly, disoriented, alone, short of breath, possible drug addict.

Mr. Spark: young, male, with swollen ankle, states he has been waiting in the ER "for hours."

Mrs. White: "bag lady" with bad body odor, was hit by bus, is bleeding, but seems oblivious, may be drunk.

Miss Teal: assertive, 35 years old, insists her arm must be x-rayed immediately.

Mr. Zale: car accident victim, no obvious bleeding but in severe pain.

Mrs. Kane: with a 6-month-old child who has high fever, with an occasional convulsion.

Dorothy X: 16-year-old, mild bleeding from self-induced efforts to abort (four months pregnant).

Working independently, please complete the following:

1. What order should be listed for the patients to be examined?
2. What was the basis of your decisions?
3. What were the values that influenced your decision?
4. What values did you consider most important?

Working in groups of five, compare your ranking of patients with classmates and discuss the similarities and differences in values that impacted on your decisions.

Values Clarification Exercise—3

Directions:
1. Read the *Code for Nurses*.
2. Label each statement in the code as a value. For example:

Statement	*Value*
The nurse provides services with respect for human dignity and the uniqueness of the client unrestricted by considerations of social or economic status, personal attributes, or the nature of health problems.	Worth and dignity of persons

3. Which of these values are most emphasized in nursing practice?
4. Which of these values are not emphasized but should be?
5. Choose the top three values that you personally hold.

CODE FOR NURSES

1. The nurse provides services with respect for human dignity and the uniqueness of the client unrestricted by considerations of social or economic status, personal attributes, or the nature of health problems.
2. The nurse safeguards the client's right to privacy by judiciously protecting information of a confidential nature.
3. The nurse acts to safeguard the client and the public when health care and safety are affected by the incompetent, unethical, or illegal practice of any person.
4. The nurse assumes responsibility and accountability for individual nursing judgments and actions.
5. The nurse maintains competence in nursing.
6. The nurse exercises informed judgment and uses individual competence and qualifications as criteria in seeking consultation, accepting responsibilities, and delegating nursing activities to others.
7. The nurse participates in activities that contribute to the ongoing development of the profession's body of knowledge.
8. The nurse participates in the profession's efforts to implement and improve standards of nursing.

9. The nurse participates in the profession's efforts to establish and maintain conditions of employment conducive to high quality nursing care.
10. The nurse participates in the profession's effort to protect the public from misinformation and misrepresentation and to maintain the integrity of nursing.
11. The nurse collaborates with members of the health professions and other citizens in promoting community and national efforts to meet the health needs of the public.

Appendix 1-B

Sample Values Inquiry Exercises

Values inquiry is a method that seeks to explore the meaning and possibilities of a human situation by discovering the values that motivate others. In contrast to values clarification, which promotes the identification and clarification of personal values, values inquiry focuses on the concept of values within social and moral issues.

The materials for values inquiry in nursing education are limitless (e.g. poems, autobiographies, biographies, novels, newspaper and magazine articles, etc.).

The only limit is the educators' own ability to link current events, literature, and other materials to classroom objectives.

Letter to a Patient

Directions:
1. The instructor requests that students write an anonymous letter to one of their patients.
2. The instructor collects all the letters and redistributes them to individual students (it is to be hoped that they do not get their own letter back).
3. Students are given the following assignment:
   - Identify the human values that are expressed in the letter (i.e., love, cooperation, acceptance, dignity, etc.).
   - Write a response to the letter.
   - Working in pairs, share your letter and response with a classmate.
   - Identify the human values that are expressed in the response.

Listening with the Third Ear, or Focus Listening

Directions:

Discussion
1. Choose a topic for discussion and have two students volunteer to discuss the subject extemporaneously for five minutes.

Quiet writing time
2. Have the students then summarize in writing, individually and quietly, what they heard and what values were present in the discussion.

Questions
3. Inform the students they may ask clarifying or extending questions to determine the accuracy of their perceptions.

4. Ask the students to reflect on the values of others and the potential actions that may result from those values.

This activity may be carried out more than once during a class, with a new topic chosen for discussion each time.

The Novel As a Values Source

Directions:
1. The instructor chooses two novels that represent a specific theme (i.e., an individual's response to illness) or a variety of themes. For example:
   - *When Bad Things Happen to Good People* by H.S. Kushner (comforting thoughts from a rabbi)
   - *A Parting Gift* by F. Sharkey, M.D. (true story of a courageous boy facing death)
2. The instructor divides the class into two groups, each reacting to a different novel.
3. The groups, after careful reading, share information about their novels.

Chapter 2

Systematic Instructional Design*

"Would you tell me, please, which way I ought to go from here?"
"That depends a good deal on where you want to go," said the Cat.
"I don't much care,—" said Alice.
"Then it doesn't matter which way you go," said the Cat.
"So long as I get somewhere," Alice added as an explanation.
"Oh, you're sure to do that," said the Cat, "if you only walk long enough."

"Lewis Carroll" in Alice In Wonderland

A systematic approach is especially well suited to nursing instruction because it encompasses not only the teaching of facts and principles but also the development of attitudes and values and permits an unlimited variety of teaching/learning situations. Most instructors have adopted a two-component system consisting of learning activities and testing. A more effective system assumes that instruction can be revised and modified. This chapter presents a systematic approach to teaching/learning and illustrates how nursing faculty members can use it to monitor the quality of their instruction.

Instructional systems models have found increasingly broad application and acceptance in education generally (Popham & Baker, 1970; Roueche & Pitman, 1972) and in medical and health-related curricula in particular (Heidgerken, 1965; Holcomb & Garner, 1973).

There are several justifications for using a systematic approach to instruction:

---

*Material in this chapter is adapted with permission from King, E.C. *Classroom evaluation strategies*. St. Louis: The C.V. Mosby Co., © 1979.

41

- to provide a more integrated, coordinated, and complete program of instruction
- to provide for consideration of individual differences such as in academic background, learning style, and previous clinical experience
- to provide competency-based instruction
- to ensure a systematic development of learning experiences through the use of appropriate teaching methods and materials
- to establish a reliable and valid means of assessment.

As nursing educators use a systematic approach to design learning experiences, they realize the benefit of integrated planning. However, other advantages also begin to emerge:

- the applicability of systematized approaches for both undergraduate and graduate nursing programs
- the desirability of changing from teaching-oriented to learning-oriented modes of instruction
- the variety of methods, materials, and assessment procedures available to expand and reinforce instruction
- the way a competency-based format of instruction contributes to a nonthreatening learning and testing environment
- the ease of identifying and measuring changes in student behavior after instruction and of documenting those changes to produce a strong statement of instructional accountability.

Many useful systems models have been developed for instructional planning. The model presented here (Figure 2-1) has been discussed extensively by Roueche and Pitman (1972) and includes as the system's components: rationale, goals and objectives, preassessment, learning strategies, postassessment, and instructional revision.

All of the elements of the model are interactive, each representing a specific task; they build on one another to create the desired change in behavior. The instructional revision component interacts throughout in a cyclical feedback process to monitor all phases of the system continuously. Other models are more complex and sophisticated, with more components and variables involved in instructional planning. However, while Figure 2-1 represents a simplistic system, it is not simple. It works as well as other, more complex models and provides the instructional planner with a basic conceptual framework that may be applied to a variety of problems.

The rest of this chapter analyzes each element of the systems model as it relates to instructional planning for nursing educators.

Figure 2-1 A Systems Model for Instruction

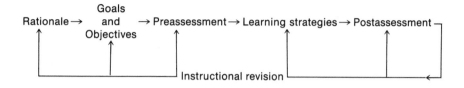

Source: Reprinted from *Classroom Evaluation Strategies* by Elizabeth C. King with permission of The C.V. Mosby Company, © 1979.

THE RATIONALE STATEMENT

A written rationale statement provides the student with some explanation or justification for studying a unit. It also gives the instructor an opportunity to explain and justify the content selected for a particular unit of study.

A rationale statement helps answer content questions students may ask:

"Why do I need to read *Stigma* by Erving Goffman? My primary goal is medical/surgical nursing?"

"Why should I study ethics? I want to be a nurse not a philosopher!"

These are not cynical questions reflecting rejection of traditional nursing instruction; rather, they are examples of student concern for relevant, significant course content. Student demands for rationale statements are valid. While pointing out important course and/or unit content, these statements also provide students with a sense of self-direction and purpose.

For example, a rationale statement for a unit on values in an approach to ethical decision making could be written as follows:

Patients' rights and responsibilities need to be considered when determining the nurse's role in patient care. A conflict of values often emerges as students prepare nursing plans over factors such as life itself as an absolute value, the quality of life, and the autonomy of the patient. To explore these conflicting values, this unit will discuss such issues as: What principles can we consider when values are in conflict? What guidelines can we use to order our thinking? How can we best weigh alternative courses of action?

GOALS AND OBJECTIVES

The first step in the identification of goals is to specify all the competencies, tasks, and responsibilities necessary for the entry-level practitioner. These competencies can be developed and validated by on-the-job task analysis and the use of advisory committees exploring such areas as: the nature of man, societal goals and trends, professional goals and trends, the nature of the learner, the nature of the teaching-learning process, and theories of nursing (Reilly, 1980). Consideration of these factors will help curriculum developers plan a nursing program with a conceptual framework that is acceptable to the entire faculty. Once overall program goals are identified, specific objectives may be developed.

A goal is a broad statement of purpose. It should represent a logical implementation of a well-defined need. Goals are not written in terms of precise, observable behavior but rather broadly describe overall learning outcomes in nonspecific terms. Sample goals statements are:

- The student will assist the patient with activities of daily living and encourage appropriate self-care.
- The student will administer medications and therapeutic treatments prescribed for the patient.
- The student will be able to recognize stresses in human relationships between patients, patients' families, visitors, and health care personnel.

These statements provide an overall description of the learning experience. A systems approach to instruction accepts goal setting as the prerequisite to effective teaching and evaluation.

In contrast to goals, objectives are more specific statements that describe observable student behavior. The key to writing objectives is to develop a basic honesty about what is required and what is not (Roueche, 1976). When instructors clearly define what they hope to accomplish, both they and their students experience minimal frustration when performance is evaluated.

Having selected specific goals for a nursing program, instructors can identify specific objectives by asking one question: When a nurse exhibits a specific competency, what is its underlying cognitive, psychomotor, and/ or affective base? The answer can be stated in terms of specific behaviors that the student should be able to exhibit. These behaviors then can be classified and sequenced. The answer also assumes a knowledge of the taxonomy or classification of behavioral objectives in three domains of learning: the cognitive, the psychomotor, and the affective.

The literature suggests two major classifications for behavioral objectives—specific and general.

Specific Behavioral Objectives

Specific behavioral objectives are especially useful for developing materials in the cognitive domain that can be adapted for programmed learning and/or independent study modules. These objectives include four major elements (Mager, 1962):

1. Audience: A description of the person(s) for whom the objective is intended.
2. Behavior: A description of the observable actions/behavior that the learner is to perform or exhibit.
3. Conditions: An outline of the conditions under which the students will perform or exhibit the actions/behavior or the factors affecting them:

   - in the classroom, laboratory, or clinical setting . . .
   - upon completion of assignment or learning task . . .
   - after reviewing instruction . . .
   - following a lecture, demonstration, or discussion . . .
   - with (without) use of notes, text, laboratory manuals . . .
   - when provided with certain materials or equipment . . .
   - given a case study, diagram, clinical problem . . .
   - on a model, classmate, patient . . .
   - given a multiple choice examination . . .
   - given a biographical data form to complete five years after graduation . . .
   - given 10 unobtrusive faculty observations
   - given a series of potential actions
   - given a film involving actions inconsistent with professional values. (Daniell, n.d.)
4. Degree: Specification of the level of achievement indicating acceptable performance:

   - to a degree of accuracy, e.g., 90 percent or $\pm$ 1 standard deviation
   - to a stated proportion, e.g., within 2 cm of mercury
   - within a given time period
   - within a given number of trials
   - to a standard of clinical acceptability
   - in accordance with recommendations or suggestions of some external organization or authority

- with verification by an external agency, panel, person
- according to criteria set forth in a laboratory manual, standard operating policy, skill analysis, or other document
- consistent with any specifiable quantity, e.g., five factors, at least two examples
- in compliance with criteria presented by the instructor (Daniell, n.d.).

An example of a specific behavioral objective is phrased as follows:

Example: "After completion of a values clarification exercise, students will be able to examine their attitudes toward physically disabled persons within an hour's time."

This then is analyzed as follows:

"After completion of a values clarification
exercise,   —CONDITION
students   —AUDIENCE
will be able to examine their attitudes toward
physically disabled persons   —BEHAVIOR
within an hour's time."   —DEGREE

General Behavioral Objectives

The guidelines for general behavioral objectives were suggested by Kibler, Barker, and Miles (1970), and Tyler (1950). There are three elements in a general behavioral objective:

1. Audience: a description of the learner
2. Behavior: a description of the observable actions/behaviors that the learner is to perform or exhibit
3. Content: a statement regarding the content to which the behavior relates.

Kibler et al. combine the description of the behavior and the content to which it relates. These also are combined when writing specific behavioral objectives.

General behavioral objectives may be analyzed as follows:

Example: "The student will respond supportively to a patient expressing grief."

"The student   —AUDIENCE
will respond supportively   —BEHAVIOR
to a patient expressing grief."   —CONTENT

Example: "The student will form judgments regarding the rights of individuals admitted to a long-term care facility."

"The student   —AUDIENCE
will form judgments   —BEHAVIOR
regarding the rights of   —CONTENT
individuals admitted to a long-
term care facility."

Both types require that the objective be written in behavioral terms; that is, a term that is observable and measurable. However, Kibler et al. caution educators against overemphasizing the action component of each objective. States of affect and cognition often are only inferred from psychomotor actions. For example, instructors do not see a student synthesize a patient care plan, they hear or read a report of it. Consequently, the significant component of the action behavior is not merely the psychomotor component but also the fact that it is somehow measurable.

Both types of objectives (general and specific) are based on the assumption that the nature of the learner must be specified, the objective must be expressed in terms of behavior, and a statement must be included regarding the content to which the conduct relates. However, general objectives do not include information regarding the conditions of learning or the performance criteria.

As mentioned earlier, specific behavioral objectives seem more appropriate for cognitive educational experiences that are adaptable to such strategies as programmed learning. In addition they may be very useful for planning for psychomotor skill learning. In contrast, general behavioral objectives are useful for communicating the basic intent of a unit, program, or course of study.

Most of the behavioral objectives in this book are general in nature. While they do not specify conditions for learning or performance criteria, they do seem appropriate for identifying affective outcomes. As such, they help inform students of expected behaviors, provide faculty members with directions for planning, and give administrators an understanding of the intent of the unit, program, or course of study.

Critics of behavioral objectives argue that actions that can be stated in behavioral terms tend not to be very important, that they limit achievement by putting ceilings on student aspirations, and that it is impossible to specify and evaluate all the outcomes that might be accomplished by instruction (Trimble, 1973).

Advocates of behavioral objectives counter with the comment that important or not, it never is possible to measure intangibles so it is far better to concentrate on the attainable. They also assert that attainment of objectives does not diminish students' aspirations but rather it motivates them. However, a third criticism, that it is impossible to evaluate all the outcomes of instruction, probably is applicable. Educators probably never can measure the total impact of the nursing curriculum on students but that criticism does not diminish the importance of defining what they are trying to accomplish.

While behaviorally stated objectives are not the panacea for curing all the ills of education, they are an attempt to initiate honest, effective communication between nursing instructors and students. They provide a direction for learning, often specify evaluation criteria, and assist instructors in testing only the content presented. While it is unlikely that objectives will proliferate to the extent recommended by some educators, teachers and students need some of the sense of direction that is provided by objectives.

DEVELOPING AFFECTIVE OBJECTIVES: A TAXONOMY

A taxonomy is a logical system for ordering behaviors within a developmental approach. Krathwohl, Bloom, and Masia (1964) provide a theoretical basis for taxonomies, a discussion of their development, and their application to educational programs. It stems from Bloom's (1956) taxonomy. They state that a taxonomy aids educators in clarifying objectives, provides a system for ordering evaluation instruments, offers a mechanism for comparing educational programs, and includes guidelines for ordering educational outcomes.

Consideration of the affective taxonomy assists nursing educators in planning experiences that not only consider awareness but also the valuing process and the internalization of values. Since educators must plan experiences that reflect the worth and dignity of each human being, they must emphasize the higher levels of the affective taxonomy in nursing programs.

The affective taxonomy represents a broad classification of human behaviors and considers a progressive developmental approach. As a hierarchical structure, each behavior builds upon a preceding one. Table 2-1 outlines the five major classes of the affective domain, gives examples of measurable behavior, and lists verbs for use in writing objectives for each class.

Table 2-1 Learning Outcomes in the Affective Domain

Class or Category	Measurable Behavior	Verbs for Writing Objectives
1.0 Receiving (being conscious of "attending to" the affective objective)	Listens attentively; attends to; demonstrates awareness, sensitivity, and interest	Listens, attends, selects, prefers, shares, accepts, describes, follows, guides, identifies, locates, names, observes, replies
2.0 Responding (implies a continuum ranging from compliance to satisfaction in response)	Participates in discussion, volunteers, acts willingly, expresses satisfaction in, is willing to support, considers opposing views	States, answers, lists, writes, develops, views, imitates, offers, shares, supports, appraises, approaches, asks, compares, contrasts, differentiates, watches, discriminates, discusses, evaluates, examines, interprets, questions, reads, recognizes, reports, reviews, selects, summarizes
3.0 Valuing (standards and patterns of choice that have worth)	Assumes responsibility, cooperates with, participates in, is convinced of, justifies role of, accepts concern for, accepts commitment to	Accepts, acclaims, agrees, assists, helps, respects, supports, participates, attains, visits, demonstrates, volunteers, attempts, joins, commits, completes, concludes, emphasizes, maintains, proposes, reports, shares, supports, verifies, persuades, defends, advocates, criticizes, approves challenge

Table 2-1 continued

Class or Category	Measurable Behavior	Verbs for Writing Objectives
4.0 Organization (conceptualization of a value system)	Uses systematic planning, practices cooperation, accepts responsibility, participates in, formulates a position, is consistent, takes a stand, serves as a model	Associates, selects, chooses, defends, challenges, advocates, assesses, criticizes, judges, approves, argues, debates, declares, defends, advises, alters, arranges, cooperates, displays, influences, initiates, organizes, practices, pursues, recommends, relates
5.0 Characterization (internal consistency of response)	Acts consistently, formulates a life plan, consistently demonstrates, serves as a model, stands for, is accountable	Adheres, combines, accepts, defends, demonstrates, exemplifies, extends, generalizes, influences, persists, practices, qualifies, reinforces, synthesizes, verifies

Source: Adapted from *Taxonomy of Educational Objectives, Handbook 2: The Affective Domain* by D.R. Krathwohl, B.S. Bloom, and B.B. Masia, published by Longman, Inc., New York, N.Y. Copyright © 1964, by permission of Longman, Inc.

The developmental process led Krathwohl and his colleagues to the principle or construct of internalization. Internalization results from an awareness of a construct or concept, then valuing that concept, and finally to internalizing the concept so that it guides personal behavior.

The principle of internalization they describe is consistent with the valuing process proposed by Raths, Harmin, & Simon (1966) discussed in Chapter 1. Both processes involve cognitive action and require the blending of intellect and emotion.

The affective taxonomy of Krathwohl et al. (1964) is outlined as follows:

1.0 Receiving (attending)
   1.1 Awareness
   1.2 Willingness to receive
   1.3 Controlled or selected attention

2.0 Responding
   2.1 Acquiescence in responding
   2.2 Willingness to respond
   2.3 Satisfaction in response
3.0 Valuing
   3.1 Acceptance of a value
   3.2 Preference for a value
   3.3 Commitment (conviction)
4.0 Organization
   4.1 Conceptualization of a value
   4.2 Organization of a value system
5.0 Characterization by a value or value complex
   5.1 Generalized set
   5.2 Characterization.

The discussion next describes each level of the affective domain, provides a sample objective, a sample activity, and a possible assessment procedure.

1.0 Receiving (Attending)

At this level, instructors are concerned that the learners merely be conscious of "attending to" the affective objective. However, this does not assume that they do not already have some personal feelings relevant to the topic under consideration. For example, previous experiences with mentally ill patients may already have affected their attitudes, values, and feelings toward the mentally ill. The Receiving category is divided into three subcategories:

1.1 Awareness

This requires that the students become merely aware or conscious of something.

Sample Objective: The students develop an awareness of the importance of respecting clients in a mental health setting.
Sample Activity: The students will read and discuss three case histories of persons who could be considered to hold positions of respect who previously have been mental patients (i.e., a physician, a member of the clergy, a professor, etc.).
Possible Assessment: The students will write a one-page discussion of the similarities and differences between the normal and abnormal behav-

iors presented in the case studies. The assessment is basically cognitive in nature. A strong cognitive base underlies the lower levels of the affective domain. This cognitive base is an essential prerequisite to influencing the valuing process.

1.2 Willingness to Receive

At the least, learners are not actively seeking to avoid the stimuli; at best, they are willing to receive or attend to them.

Sample Objective: The students acknowledge the rights of mental patients.
Sample Activity: The students will read the *Standards for Nursing Practice* proposed by the American Nurses' Association (1976).
Possible Assessment: The students will write a response to an essay question relating the rights of mental patients to the standards for nursing practice. This still is the receiving level and the students basically are receiving cognitive information. For an in-depth discussion of writing and scoring the essay question, see the section in Chapter 4 on "Adapting Traditional Evaluation Methods to Assessing Affective Objectives."

1.3 Controlled or Selected Attention

In contrast to greater instructor control in the previous levels, this stage contains an element of the learner's controlling the situation so that the student selects the desired stimulus despite competing stimuli.

Sample Objective: The nursing students actively listen to all patients to whom they are assigned.
Sample Activity: The students, while providing nursing care, stop to listen when appropriate.
Possible Assessment: Rating Scale for Listening Skills (Exhibit 2-1).

Exhibit 2-1 Rating Scale for Listening Skills

0 = Inattentive listener. Little or no eye contact. Does not look at patient talking. Appears absorbed in procedure only.

1 = Partially attentive listener. Minimal eye contact but primarily focuses on the procedure, not the patient.

2 = Frequently maintains appropriate eye contact while listening to patient. Acceptable focus on both patient and procedure.

3 = Consistently maintains appropriate eye contact while listening to patient. Demonstrates exceptional awareness of the need to listen and complete the procedure simultaneously.

2.0 Responding

Responding goes one step beyond merely attending to a situation; it implies a continuum of responding ranging from compliance through requiring some degree of satisfaction in response.

2.1 Acquiescence in Responding

The term "compliance" often is used to describe this behavior. While the students may make the response, they have not fully accepted the rationale for it. While compliance objectives are not ideal targets, goals relative to health and safety can be found at this level.

An issue often discussed regarding "acquiescence" in responding is that while reacting or answering in such a manner may have the same external conduct as internalized behavior, the latter is different.

Sample Objective: The nursing students will read a biography of an individual who has experienced mental illness.
Sample Activity: The students will choose a biography/autobiography of their choice of an individual who has experienced mental illness.
Sample Assessment: The students will summarize the biography in no more than two pages.

2.2 Willingness to Respond

This is an important category for educational objectives for it implies a "willingness" or voluntary response from free choice. As a result, many of the affective objectives at this level are desirable. In fact, once the students begin exhibiting the appropriate behaviors, the environment often provides reinforcement that will guarantee continuation of such conduct. Consequently the instructor's task often is only to provide the appropriate environment.

Sample Objective: The nursing students willingly seek opportunities to be of service to mental health patients.
Sample Activity: The students voluntarily organize a social affair for a small group of patients.
Sample Assessment: Each student will develop an anecdotal record such as in Exhibit 2-2. (For a more complete description of writing anecdotal records, see Chapter 4.)

2.3 Satisfaction in Response

Many educational objectives are found at this level. Not only are the students "willing to respond" but their behavior is followed by feelings

Exhibit 2-2 Example of an Anecdotal Record

Date: 2/23/83

Observer: Anne A.

Description of Incident: Susan voluntarily organized a trip to the farmers market for four mental patients—Bill, Carol, Tim, and Janet. When they returned they prepared fresh fruit and vegetable salads. Susan was heard saying, "This has been a very good day. Bill cooked and ate fresh asparagus for the first time and Janet seemed less withdrawn than usual."

Comment: Susan seemed to enjoy planning the trip and was happy with the outcome.

---

of pleasure and/or satisfaction. This internalized feeling serves as an intrinsic reward that tends to increase the frequency of the behavior. Obviously this focuses on the emotional component and its importance in learning.

Sample Objective: The nursing students take pleasure in planning leisure activities with mental health patients.

Sample Activity: The students conduct a survey to assess patients' leisure time interests.

Sample Assessment: Use open-ended items as a projective technique, as in Exhibit 2-3.

The first two levels of the affective taxonomy, as noted, consider value indicators. The affective responses of receiving and reading that are elicited do not meet all seven criteria of the valuing process and thus cannot be considered values. Raths et al. (1966) suggest these may be potential values and refer to them as value indicators. These may include aspirations, attitudes, interests, feelings, beliefs, and/or convictions.

Exhibit 2-3 Open-Ended Items as a Projective Technique

---

1. Some of the patients here want to _____.
2. If given the opportunity I like to plan for _____.
3. In working with other people I _____.
4. Someone who is very friendly and enjoys planning leisure time activities for patients is _____.
5. Planning leisure time activities for the patients gave me _____.

Educators also should be cautioned that when goals are written for the first two levels, they may not be identifiable as discrete affective objectives. However, when they are viewed as a continuum within a developmental process it becomes apparent that the instructors are seeking to influence the affective domain.

At the third level, valuing, the individual makes a choice and the internalization process begins.

3.0 Valuing

Valuing implies that a thing, phenomenon, or behavior has worth. Many affective objectives are written for this level. Objectives that represent desirable outcomes as the result of the socialization process are classified here. Instructors attempt to model overt socially accepted and highly valued behaviors. As these overt behaviors are displayed and/or imitated by the students, the instructors provide reinforcement. An essential element of the behavior characterized by valuing is that it is determined by a person's internal commitment to the value and not by compliance.

Obviously the students may conform externally to socially accepted behaviors when they have only partially internalized the attitude, value, or feeling being expressed. As a result, the difficulty of measuring the congruence between intrinsic feelings and external behavior is a challenge.

Values can be defined as standards and patterns of choice that guide persons and groups toward satisfaction, fulfillment, and meaning. Raths et al. stress that holding a value involves an active process of choosing and prizing personal beliefs and acting on them. For a value to be present there must be some overt behavior that demonstrates that value. Mature, developed, internalized patterns of behavior are consistent in several different situations. Values exist as standards for action. Consequently, values never are actualized fully except as they orient choice and shape conduct (Morrill, 1980).

3.1 Acceptance of a Value

At this level the students are so consistent in describing the worth of a behavior that observers can identify the value. Furthermore, the students are willing to be identified with the value.

Sample Objective: The nursing students demonstrate a sense of responsibility for promoting quality nursing care for mental patients.
Sample Activity: The students read a case study and determine the position and action they will take.

Sample Situation: You are one of two night staff nurses in a private psychiatric hospital. A 19-year-old female who is a previous patient and a known drug abuser is admitted. She is not oriented to time and place but can state her name. She mumbles, "I want to live with mother. No, I want to live with daddy." After a brief assessment, Marilyn, the other night staff nurse, takes an unscheduled coffee break and leaves you to care for all the patients. When Marilyn returns, you ask her to recheck the patient as she is not as verbal as she was upon admission. Forty-five minutes later when you ask how the patient is doing, Marilyn replies, "She's stopped rambling about her mother and daddy. I hope she stays quiet until the doctor arrives." You recheck the patient yourself and note all vital signs are depressed. Marilyn appears and observes you recording the vital signs. You share your results with her and she says, "I was just going to check her." What action would you take regarding Marilyn's behavior? Share your action with the class.

Sample Assessment: The students relate Marilyn's actions to Kohlberg's (1975) stages of moral development (see Chapter 1).

3.2 Preference for a Value

This level implies not just acceptance of a value but sufficient commitment to pursue it actively.

Sample Objective: The nursing students assume responsibility for influencing federal legislation relevant to mental health.

Sample Activity: The students write letters to local, state, and federal service agencies regarding the deinstitutionalization of mental health patients.

Possible Assessment: The students develop, implement, and analyze a value activities program (Exhibit 2-4).

3.3 Commitment

At this level there is an emotional acceptance of the belief. Individuals not only model acceptance of their belief but strive to convince others and actively seek converts to it. Consequently, characteristics that are essential to commitments are that (1) the value must endure over a period of time and (2) there must be an investment of personal energy in the attitude or belief that is held.

Sample Objective: The nursing students educate others concerning the capabilities and needs of the mentally ill patient.

Sample Activity: The students plan continuing inservice education programs concerning mental illness.

Exhibit 2-4 A Value Activities Program

Instructions: For each of the following activities circle: O = if you perform the activity occasionally F = if you perform the activity frequently N = if you never perform the activity			

1. Attend public meetings regarding issues relevant
   to mental health.   O   F   N
2. Write letters attempting to influence federal
   legislation involving mental health.   O   F   N
3. Plan education programs concerning mental illness.   O   F   N
4. Disseminate current research articles to peers
   regarding psychotropic drugs.   O   F   N
5. Volunteer to coordinate a field trip for mental
   health patients.   O   F   N

Possible Assessment: Developing evaluation strategies for this third level is difficult because instructors must strive to document consistent standards and patterns of human behavior. However, a variety of observation assessment forms may be useful, such as rating scales, checklists, and anecdotal records. Their development is discussed in Chapter 4.

4.0 Organization

Organization is defined as the conceptualization and classification of a value system.

4.1 Conceptualization of a Value

During the conceptualization process, students begin to see how the value relates to those they already hold or to new ones they are coming to hold.

Sample Objective: The nursing students form judgments as to the responsibility of society for the proper treatment of mental health patients.
Sample Activity: The students hold a group discussion that includes evidence of abstract thinking concerning the following situation.
Situation: For the last five days, you have been caring for a 32-year-old mother of three who is hospitalized with a nonspecific diagnosis of a personality disorder. She was accompanied by her husband upon admis-

sion. She asks constantly to see him but he has yet to visit the patient. You call the husband and explain the wife's requests for a visit. He replies that he does not have time for any visits, that his wife's hospitalization has provided him with an opportunity to finish some work. He requests you to tell his wife to "Hang in there!"
Possible Assessment: The students assume they were the staff nurse in that situation and describe what action they would take regarding the husband's behavior. Each nursing student shares that individual plan of action with the class and relates it to the problem-solving process.

Again, the instructor should be aware of the limitations of the assessment process for this level of the affective domain, where there is a strong interdependence between knowledge and responsibility. The conceptualization of a value requires the students to act upon those values. There will be opportunities to act upon values during the clinical education component of the curriculum.

4.2 Organization of a Value System

This requires the students to reduce the cognitive dissonance regarding the value and to bring seemingly conflicting values into an ordered relationship.

Sample Objective: The nursing students weigh alternative social policies and practices for caring for the mentally ill against traditional ones.
Sample Activity: Each student writes a research paper that traces the history of medical care for the mentally ill, comparing contemporary traditional practices with alternative practices. They then recommend their own suggestions for patient care plans.
Evaluation: Critical analysis of the research paper.

5.0 Characterization by a Value or Value Complex

Rarely, if ever, are the goals of education set at this level of the affective domain. Realistically, formal education cannot reach this level, where the relationship between cognitive and affective processes becomes pronounced and integrated. Arriving at this level takes considerable time, possibly a life time. Consequently, the brief time of an academic program would not be sufficient to accomplish objectives at this level. An individual arriving at this level has done so through painful intellectual effort (Krathwohl et al., 1964).

At this level of internalization of value(s), the individual's behavior is consistent with the value(s) held and the person has integrated them into a personal philosophy of life.

5.1 Generalized Set

Generalized set is a consistent response to related situations that provides internal consistency to the system of attitudes and values held. It is selective generalized responding at a very high level.

5.2 Characterization

This involves a value system whereby individuals develop a consistent philosophy of life. In a sense it may be described as maturity.

Sample Objective: The nursing students develop a consistent philosophy of life, viewing problems in objective, realistic, and tolerant terms.
Sample Activity: The students write responses to letters to the editor regarding situations related to respect for mental health patients as in Exhibit 2-5.
Evaluation: In reality it is very difficult if not impossible to evaluate this level of the affective domain. The instructor may be able to identify critical incidents that reflect the behavior in the sample objective but evaluation in the traditional sense is probably not possible.

Exhibit 2-5 Example of a Characterization Value Activity

Directions:
The instructor comments to the students: "The following letter to the editor raises some interesting points. Write a response, using factual information relating to group homes. I will pick one of your responses to send to the editor. See your name in print!"

Dear Editor: It seems that some politicians will do anything to get votes. The recommendation to establish a group home for deinstitutionalized mental patients in my neighborhood is untenable. We will have to live in constant fear, with our doors locked at all times. Our property values will decrease. The patients will be a physical and psychological threat to our children, limiting their freedom of play. If the politicians believe we need more "crazy" houses why don't they locate them in their own neighborhoods?

P.R.K.
New York, New York

Again, instructors should be aware of the limitations of planning educational experiences and evaluation strategies for this level of the affective domain because the students will be at various stages of the internalization process, many of them just developing their value systems. However, instructors must help provide settings for them to act upon their beliefs, for it is only through this personal action that values can develop fully.

Educators should use their affective objectives and their resultant assessment procedures only as guidelines for behavior while being ever cognizant of their inherent weaknesses. While there are difficulties in stating and assessing affective outcomes, they are most important in providing a total educational experience for students. Instructors' values and attitudes are showing all during classroom and clinical teaching experiences. However crude their efforts to teach and assess affective learning, each attempt will provide new ideas and directions for others.

PREASSESSMENT OF STUDENTS' LEARNING

Students' prior education always affects the way they achieve new learning. Consequently, to develop the most effective teaching/learning sequences, instructors must determine what knowledge, skills, attitudes, and values the nursing students bring to the classroom and/or clinical setting. Instruction simply cannot accommodate differences if it cannot distinguish them.

Preassessment is a check on the current state of the students' knowledge and skill in reference to a planned future status. In practice, preassessment often is merely a verbal check; at times, this may be sufficient. However, nothing can take the place of thorough knowledge of students' abilities, skills, attitudes, and values before instruction begins.

The best way instructors can determine whether students can perform a psychomotor task is to have them actually do it; to preassess cognitive information, a written pretest often is recommended. In addition, there are a variety of assessment techniques that can be used to preassess attitudes and values. (Chapter 4 describes the development of three commonly used assessment scales.) Table 2-2 provides an example of planning for preassessment (Wong & Raulerson, 1974). Two examples of preassessment strategies for the objective written in Table 2-2 are presented in Exhibit 2-6.

Instructors should remember that Semantic Differential Scales at best measure only general impressions. They may be useful when it is suspected that individuals hold strong emotional feelings about attitudes or objects but lack a well-developed knowledge base. For a more complete discussion of assessing attitudes, see Chapter 4.

Table 2-2 Flow Diagram for Preassessment

Assume All Know	Preassess	Objective
Etiology, signs, and symptoms of mental illness $\rightarrow$	Current attitudes toward the mentally ill $\rightarrow$	Given at least ten unobtrusive faculty observations over a two-semester period in the clinical setting, the student will demonstrate positive attitudes toward working with the mentally ill.

Source: Adapted from *A Guide to Instructional Design* by M.R. Wong and J.D. Raulerson, published by Educational Technology Publications, Inc., Englewood Cliffs, N.J. Copyright © 1974, by permission of Educational Technology Publications, Inc.

Exhibit 2-6 Two Sample Preassessment Strategies

EXAMPLE 1.

A suggested technique for assessing a generalized attitude objective that may be used before and after psychiatric nursing is the Semantic Differential Scale developed by Osgood, Suci, and Tannenbaum (1957). The assessment instrument takes the form of a rating scale of bipolar adjective pairs related to the concept of the attitude(s) of interest to the instructor. Students check the scale value along the adjective continuum corresponding with their first impression toward the concept in question.

Directions:
Please respond with your first impression. Below are suggested guidelines for each scale position.

Concept

polar term (X)   __:__:__:__:__:__:__: polar term (Y)

        1   2   3   4   5   6   7

1 = extremely X	4 = neither X nor Y	5 = slightly Y
2 = quite X		6 = quite Y
3 = slightly X		7 = extremely Y

Mentally Ill Patients

fierce	__:__:__:__:__:__:	gentle
ugly	__:__:__:__:__:__:	beautiful
clean	__:__:__:__:__:__:	dirty
valuable	__:__:__:__:__:__:	worthless
pleasant	__:__:__:__:__:__:	unpleasant
good	__:__:__:__:__:__:	bad
harmless	__:__:__:__:__:__:	harmful

Exhibit 2-6 continued

EXAMPLE 2.

A preassessment and postassessment instrument may be constructed to determine attitudes toward the mentally ill before and after the course of study.

Directions:
Circle how much you agree or disagree with the following statements.*

SA = Strongly Agree
A = Agree
U = Undecided
D = Disagree
SD = Strongly Disagree

1. Mentally ill patients cannot expect to lead a completely full or satisfying life. SA A U D SD
2. It is a mistake for mentally ill patients to marry. SA A U D SD
3. Mentally ill patients can and do learn things all the time. SA A U D SD
4. Cities should reserve apartments in regular housing for deinstitutionalized mental patients. SA A U D SD
5. Some physical exercise is good for the mentally ill. SA A U D SD
6. Work is often good for the mentally ill. SA A U D SD
7. Former mental health patients should be allowed to fill leadership positions. SA A U D SD
8. All mentally ill patients should be institutionalized. SA A U D SD
9. All mentally ill patients are dangerous to others. SA A U D SD
10. Mentally ill patients can get well. SA A U D SD

Note: A more complete description of this technique is included in Chapter 4 with directions for scoring.

*The attitude scale is a sample written by the author for illustrative purposes only.

Now that the course objective has been written and a preassessment has been conducted, the instructor can begin to develop appropriate learning strategies.

LEARNING STRATEGIES

Planning for the presentation of content requires integration of the decisions about the selection of appropriate teaching methods and media.

Teaching Methods

Several guidelines may be considered when determining appropriate teaching methods.

First, the teaching method must be suited to the objectives and the content characteristics. Depending on the objectives to be met, certain instructional methods may be superior. Davies (1973), summarizing the research literature, suggests the following generalizations in choosing an appropriate teaching method:

> All teaching strategies can be used to accomplish cognitive objectives. However, lower-order cognitive objectives can best be accomplished by lecture, lecture-discussion, programmed instruction, and computer-assisted instruction and higher-order cognitive objectives can be accomplished by all teaching strategies. Lower-order affective objectives (those emphasizing receiving, responding, valuing) can be effectively taught by utilizing all teaching strategies. Higher-order affective objectives (those emphasizing organizing and internalizing) can be most effectively taught by group discussion, role playing, case studies, leaderless groups, and sensitivity training.
>
> Psychomotor objectives are best accomplished by lecture-demonstration, practical tutorials, and independent study with practice.

Second, the instructor must have knowledge of learning and motivational theory before choosing a particular teaching method. The following principles of learning and motivation are brief statements derived from the writings of learning theorists. These principles should be considered before selection of a teaching method.

- *Students are likely to be motivated to learn things that are meaningful* (Ausubel, 1968). Ausubel argues that new material must relate to information the student already possesses. When new material is related to previously acquired knowledge, the new information is remembered more easily.

- *Students are more likely to learn something new if they have all the prerequisites* (Ausubel, 1968; Gagne, 1970). Ausubel emphasizes the necessity for student mastery of previous knowledge before new information is given. Furthermore, Ausubel suggests that the weak predictive validity of some pretests is a direct result of the inadequate estimate of students' prior cognitive knowledge. Similarly, Gagne recommends that before teaching new tasks, the instructor should ensure that all prerequisite ones have been mastered.

- *Students are more likely to acquire new behavior if they are presented with a model performance to watch and imitate* (Bandura & Walters, 1963). Perhaps the greatest advantage of learning by imitation is that it provides a complete behavioral sequence for the student.
- *Students are more likely to learn by novel presentations* (Ausubel, 1968). In Ausubel's system, the ability to remember is a function of whether or not the new information can be dissociated from existing material. Consequently, if new material is very similar to what exists, it tends to be forgotten more quickly; if it is an extension of existing material but novel, it will be remembered longer.
- *Students are more likely to learn if instructional conditions are made pleasant* (Skinner, 1969). Skinner argues that much of current educational practice is based on aversive control that is used for both disciplinary and instructional purposes. He recommends positive reinforcement of desired behavior and ignoring of undesirable conduct as the means of producing a warmer and more rewarding classroom environment. Instructors should do as much as they can to send away as many students as possible with good feelings about the class.
- *Students are more likely to learn if they are actively involved in the instructional process* (Bandura & Walters, 1963). Active involvement is more effective than mere observation. The opportunity to apply new knowledge actively is essential to success in learning and to increased retention. Active involvement in the learning process is critical to the development of psychomotor skills.
- *The teaching/learning experience must provide the necessary conditions for the transfer of knowledge* (Bruner, 1966). Bruner encourages instructors to develop exercises and learning conditions that will facilitate student discovery of the conceptual linkage between events. This linkage will maximize the possibility of the transfer of learning.
- *The instructor should consider the learning style preferences of students when choosing an appropriate teaching method.* The *Canfield-Lafferty Learning Styles Inventory* yields data that can be useful to nursing instructors (Canfield, 1974). Instructors can determine the students' preferred learning styles and use this information to avoid imposing their own preferences on the class. More importantly, the *Learning Styles Inventory* can be used to determine preferences of individual students and groups. With this information, the instructor can develop a variety of classroom and clinical experiences to reach the maximum number of students. It has been suggested that *Learning Styles Inventory* results be used to match students and teachers. However, with the limited supply of nursing educators, this seems

unrealistic. Just possibly the educational environment might be enriched by these differences.

- *The teaching method should be cost effective.* For example, some students may prefer small-group seminars but these obviously are not as cost effective as the lecture method. Clinical education is very expensive in terms of time, supplies, and personnel involved. However, it is a critical component of any nursing program because of the higher level learning involved, including the application, analysis, synthesis, and evaluation of knowledge; and the demonstration and practice of psychomotor skills and of affective learning appropriate for the clinical setting.

Any adequate discussion of the systems approach must consider teaching methods. The lecture, demonstration, laboratory method, independent study, and individualized instruction (autotutorial, programmed, and computer-assisted) are useful for the lower levels of the affective domain. However, the teaching strategies most useful for higher level affective learning include role playing, simulated gaming, group discussion, case studies, leaderless groups, and sensitivity training. Teaching methods most useful for higher level affective learning are discussed in Chapter 3.

MEDIA FOR INSTRUCTIONAL USE

Media can be grouped into six classes: print, audio, still visuals, motion visuals, human interactions, and concrete objects. In selecting which to use, the characteristics of the learner, the task, course objectives, content characteristics, and the media all must be considered.

Historically, nursing instructors and textbooks have been the media of choice, with audio or visual aids in limited use. However, the variety of media readily available is considerable. Table 2-3 suggests media choices categorically by student response modality (i.e., listening/viewing, reading, and interacting).

In determining the appropriateness of audiovisual aids, Davies (1973), after reviewing the research, concludes that they can be effective in learning. Furthermore, learning can be enhanced if instructors (1) state the objectives to be met by the media, (2) encourage student participation, and (3) use the media to repeat and reinforce previously learned information.

The medium selected should depend on the learning objectives to be met. Davies summarizes major trends and concludes that:

Table 2-3 Media Categorized by Student Response Modality

Listening/Viewing	Reading	Interacting
Audiotape	Book	Skill practice
Slidetape	Periodical	Problem solving
Videotape, film	Programmed instruction	Question exercises
Demonstration	Chalkboard	Experiments
Concrete objects	Study guide, case study	Computer-assisted instruction

Source: Reprinted from *Classroom Evaluation Strategies* by Elizabeth C. King with permission of The C.V. Mosby Company, © 1979.

- Cognitive objectives can be attained using all types of audiovisual aids.
- Affective objectives can be achieved most successfully through the use of still pictures, films, television, and audio aids.
- Psychomotor objectives can be achieved most successfully through the use of audio aids, actual manipulation of real equipment, and field trips.

In selecting a medium, the instructors also should keep in mind the principles of learning. Appropriate media will aid in the transfer of learning; provide reinforcement of the knowledge, skills, and attitudes to be acquired; and assist in retention of knowledge.

Appropriate learning strategies that incorporate the selection of methods and media can enhance instruction.

POSTASSESSMENT OF BEHAVIORAL CHANGES

Postassessment is simply the means by which quantitative changes in behavior are observed with some degree of accuracy. The central questions are: (1) What changes in behavior took place as a result of instruction? (2) How can these changes be measured? The value of educational measurement depends on the validity of the answers.

Assessment provides directions for restating objectives as well as replanning preassessment instruments and learning strategies. In this broad interpretation, all the functions of postassessment are concerned with the facilitation of learning.

In the systems model, educational measurement is conceived of as an integral part of instruction, not as a process apart from instruction. Without adequate postassessment, instructors have no way of validating judgments regarding the selection of objectives and learning strategies.

Postassessment can facilitate learning when the following conditions are met:

- The outcomes selected for testing mirror the stated objectives of the nursing program. For example, if the instructional unit focuses on problem solving in nursing practice, the testing program must measure the student's ability to solve problems. There must be a clear relationship among the level of the objective, the type of learning experience provided, and the type of measurement. (This is discussed more fully in Chapter 4.)
- Achievement testing is planned and developed as an integral part of the program of curriculum and instruction. When tests are selected and constructed in terms of the learning program, with the results used to provide immediate feedback for instructional revision, their value cannot be questioned. In contrast, testing may be viewed with suspicion when it occurs merely as a parallel activity to instruction.
- Nursing instructors take an active role in the construction and development of all tests. That puts the testing program under the direction and control of those responsible for instruction.

Postassessment can have a profound influence on the improvement of instruction but to do so, it must be seen as an integral part of the teaching/learning system and the results must be used continuously to guide changes.

Perhaps the most important outcome of evaluation is that it enables instructors to identify with some confidence the strengths and weaknesses of the teaching and learning and to plan changes in the system to correct the weaknesses.

INSTRUCTIONAL REVISION

The goal of nursing education is the attainment of specified outcomes—skills, knowledge, and attitudes. To accomplish these outcomes, strategies must be developed that identify weaknesses in teaching and learning. More importantly, educators must be able to begin again, and be committed to doing so if necessary. They must be open and flexible to change—not just for the sake of change but rather planned change based on reliable findings. As instructors recycle what was successful and discard what was not, they continually contribute to a nursing education program with sound objectives, effective teaching strategies, and competent entry level professionals.

REFERENCES

Ausubel, D.P. *Educational psychology: A cognitive view.* New York: Holt, Rinehart & Winston, Inc., 1968.

Bandura, A., & Walters, R. *Social learning and personality development.* New York: Holt, Rinehart & Winston, Inc., 1963.

Bruner, J.S. *Toward a theory of instruction.* Cambridge, Mass.: Harvard University Press, 1966.

Canfield, A.A. The Canfield-Lafferty learning styles inventory: A status report. In M.K. Morgan, C.S. Broward, & D.M. Filson (Eds.), *Cognitive and affective dimensions in health related education.* Gainesville, Fla.: Center for Allied Health Instructional Personnel, 1974.

Daniell, E., Principal developer. Instructional objectives. Teaching Improvement Project System (TIPS), Center for Learning Resources, College of Allied Health Professions, University of Kentucky, Lexington, Kentucky, n.d.

Davies, I.K. *Competency based learning: Technology, management and design.* New York: McGraw-Hill Book Company, 1973.

Gagne, R.M. *The conditions of learning* (2nd ed.). New York: Holt, Rinehart & Winston, Inc., 1970.

Heidgerken, L.E. *Teaching and learning in schools of nursing: Principles and methods.* Philadelphia: J.B. Lippincott Co., 1965.

Holcomb, J.D., & Garner, A.E. *Improving teaching in medical schools: A practical handbook.* Springfield, Ill.: Charles C Thomas, Publisher, 1973.

Kibler, R.J.; Barker, L.L.; & Miles, D.T. *Behavioral objectives and instruction.* Boston: Allyn & Bacon, Inc., 1970.

Kohlberg, L. The cognitive-developmental approach to moral education. *Phi Delta Kappan,* June 1975, *56*(1), 670-677.

Krathwohl, D.R.; Bloom, B.S.; & Masia, B.B. *Taxonomy of educational objectives, Handbook II: The affective domain.* New York: Longman, Inc., 1964.

Mager, R.F. *Preparing instructional objectives.* Belmont, Calif.: Fearon Publishers, Inc., 1962.

Morrill, R.L. *Teaching values in college.* San Francisco: Jossey-Bass, Inc., Publishers, 1980.

Osgood, C.E.; Suci, G.J.; & Tannenbaum, P.H. *The measurement of meaning.* Urbana, Ill., The University of Illinois Press, 1957.

Popham, W.J., & Baker, E.L. *Systematic instruction.* Englewood Cliffs, N.J.: Prentice-Hall, Inc., 1970.

Raths, L.E.; Harmin M.; Simon, S.B. *Values and teaching.* Columbus, Ohio: The Charles E. Merrill Publishing Co., Inc., 1966.

Reilly, D.E. *Behavioral objectives: Evaluation in nursing* (2nd ed.). New York: Appleton-Century-Crofts, Inc., 1980.

Roueche, J.E. A place to begin: A systems approach to instruction. In C.W. Ford & M.K. Morgan (Eds.), *Teaching in the health professions*. St. Louis: The C.V. Mosby Company, 1976.

Roueche, J.E., & Pitman, J. *A modest proposal: Students can learn*. San Francisco: Jossey-Bass, Inc., 1972.

Skinner, B.F. *Contingencies of reinforcement*. New York: Appleton-Century-Crofts, Inc., 1969.

Standards for nursing practice. Kansas City, Mo.: American Nurses' Association, Inc., 1976.

Trimble, W. Rabid innovators: The behavioral objectivists. *Community College Review*, July–August 1973, *1*(2), 37-41.

Tyler, R.W. *Basic principles of curriculum and instruction*. Chicago: The University of Chicago Press, 1950.

Wong, M.R., & Raulerson, J.D. *A guide to instructional design*. Englewood Cliffs, N.J.: Educational Technology Publications, Inc., 1974.

Chapter 3

Classroom Teaching Strategies

To teach is to sensitize. To words. To problems. To ideas. To anguish and humanity. Anguish is a strong word, but there is much anguish in the world. And humanity is what you do in response to anguish.

Samuel G. Freedman

The focus of this chapter is on four classroom teaching strategies for affective education: (1) group discussion, (2) the case study method, (3) role playing, and (4) simulation gaming. For each strategy, the discussion includes a definition, purposes, factors to consider when planning, a recommended procedure, and the benefits and limitations of the method. Sample case studies, role-playing exercises, and a simulated game also are presented.

GROUP DISCUSSION

Discussion is an instructional methodology in which a verbal exchange of ideas, points of view, elements of subject matter, and perceptions are shared by two or more individuals to clarify the topic under study (Maley, 1978).

Group discussion is a teaching method best used to develop both depth and breadth of knowledge. It is not generally recommended for use in presenting new material but it is effective for changing attitudes, values, and behaviors. Its use often improves students' attitudes toward their instructor and their peers. Discussion also can strengthen the students' ability to (1) participate in the free exchange of ideas; (2) express personal

71

attitudes, feelings, and beliefs; and (3) develop a logical verbal presentation of ideas. If the instructor uses effective reinforcement during a discussion, it may contribute to the students' formation of a strong self-concept. Such affective development may be characterized by a process of internalization in which the discussion leads to a strengthened perception of the inner self (Maley, 1978).

Factors in Planning To Use Discussion

Objectives

Objectives for the discussion method include problem solving; cross-peer learning; increased sensitivity to complex issues; and the clarification of attitudes, values, and beliefs (Barnes-McConnell, 1978). Alexander and Abramson (1975) state that increasing interpersonal skills, modifying opinions, and applying course content also are appropriate objectives.

Objectives that may be accomplished by the discussion method are that the nursing student will be able to:

- form judgments regarding the constitutional rights of mentally retarded patients
- examine various points of view on abortion with the intent of declaring a personal position
- express personal feelings about the ways selected individuals respond to stress
- explore personal values concerning the relationship of death to age and cause
- examine personal feelings about the sexuality of the elderly
- share experiences interacting with parents during the pediatric rotation
- formulate judgments concerning extraordinary means of maintaining life for a critically ill patient
- listen actively to peers as they express ideas for plans of care.

Group Size and Mix

Group size and mix are important factors when considering the discussion method. While 15 to 20 students is an ideal number, larger groups (i.e., 50 to 100) can be broken down into several small groups if space and furniture are appropriate.

Space and Time

Informality and freedom of movement facilitate the discussion method, so movable chairs are recommended. In addition, it is important to plan for an adequate amount of time to allow for in-depth discussion. Students should be as comfortable as possible. They should be arranged facing each other. A semicircle is a good physical arrangement. The instructor also should be able to have a face-to-face view of each student.

Instructor's Attitude and Behavior

A successful discussion leader is a supportive, open instructor who can create a basic foundation of trust within the group. This foundation of trust will support an atmosphere of mutual inquiry in which all ideas are considered important and each student is an essential member of the group.

The instructor's willingness to engage in "self-disclosure" will help lend an intimacy that otherwise might be difficult to achieve. For example, relevant experiences from an instructor's own clinical education, a difficult time, or an incident in the teacher's life that helps illustrate a concept or theory can help meet the educational objectives. Self-disclosure can convey the relevance of course material to everyday life. For example, the instructor's following personal anecdote was shared during a discussion class to help meet the objective: "The nursing student will be able to effectively counsel family members of the patient with a cardiovascular accident" (CVA).

My father had suffered a massive CVA and was hospitalized at a large tertiary care hospital. My younger brother went to visit him for the first time. The nurse told him the room and bed number for our father. My brother went to the room and returned to the nurse saying, "You must have given me the wrong room number, my father is not there." What supportive responses can the nurse offer when a son viewing a seriously ill father does not recognize him?

While it takes personal courage to tell students of past hurts, frustrations, and pain, such sharing can maximize the potential of the role model in their academic lives. A great deal of failure seems to be part of the success process. The sharing of this "failure" can support students' motivation and growth and encourage the highly successful ones as well as stimulate discussions.

Procedure for Conducting a Discussion

Group discussions often are characterized by lack of direction. To help avoid this, some procedure must be developed to help discuss the material adequately. *The Group Cognitive Map* (Hill, 1977) is a procedural tool that outlines an orderly sequence a group may follow to maximize the benefits of this teaching strategy. Use of *The Group Cognitive Map* assumes everyone has read all the required materials before the discussion; pooling ignorance is not group discussion. The steps in the *Group Cognitive Map* (Hill, 1977) are outlined in Table 3-1.

Successful classroom discussions result when the instructor has been successful in "community building," based on encouraging attitudes of concern and unconditional positive regard. Community building results when there is a genuine group cohesiveness and rapport among students and faculty that allows them to trust one another. Building community helps fill basic human needs for security, respect, self-esteem, and belonging in contrast to anxiety, hostility, self-doubt, and rejection.

In a community, students share influence with each other and the teacher, support the goals of the class, and accept individual differences. Furthermore there is a belief that shared responsibility does not exclude individuals' right to withhold their thoughts and ideas. The right to refrain from participating thus must be respected and reinforced.

Guidelines for Effective Discussions

Listen very carefully to questions since many contain an underlying statement.

Many simple questions really are statements in disguise. For example, the person who asks, "What would you do if you were told you were carrying a Down's syndrome child?" may really be saying, "I want you to commit yourself first before I disclose my true feelings," or "I'm really unsure of my feelings about mental retardation," or "I would like to have a child but because of my age, I'm worried about Down's syndrome." Since many statements are phrased as questions, it is essential to listen for those that might reflect an underlying concern that is not expressed directly.

Do not make statements that force a value judgment or position on others.

"We can all agree that terminally ill patients should volunteer to test new drugs or new medical procedures." This verbal strong-arm tactic may

Table 3-1 Steps in Cognitive Group Map

Step	*Name*	*Rationale and Behavior*
1.	Definition of terms and concepts	Mastering technical language is an objective of nursing courses. For this step the instructor may wish to have medical dictionaries available.
2.	General statement of author's message	This step provides a verbal abstract of the overall message(s) of the author(s).
3.	Identification of major themes or subtopics	This step provides an analysis of the material and its constituent elements. The analysis clarifies the relative hierarchy of ideas and communication and indicates how the latter is organized.
4.	Allocation of time	This is a crucial step. Time limits set by group consensus can help ensure both depth and breadth of coverage. The instructor must be prepared to monitor the allocation of time, no easy task.
5.	Discussion of major themes	The emphasis is completely on a full discussion of the author's message(s) and not on personal opinions of group members. This is not to devalue personal opinions but rather to focus on what authorities in a field are saying. This important step often is bypassed in group discussions. If it is skipped, a discussion on, for example, unionization of nurses may degenerate into personal opinions that lead to diversions and disagreement before the history, rationale, and pros and cons of the topic have been explored.
6.	Integration of material with other knowledge	This step requires group members to make a conscious effort to transfer principles and concepts acquired in previous learning to a new situation.
7.	Application of the material	Similar to Step 6, this one requires members to make a conscious effort to assess the possible applications and implications of the material.

Table 3-1 continued

Step	Name	Rationale and Behavior
8.	Evaluation of the author's presentation	This step finally allows students to voice their personal opinions and reactions. The previous steps have aided them in the development of critical thinking and may have helped decrease affective loading.
9.	Evaluation of group and individual performances	This step is necessary if discussion is to continue successfully. A knowledge of group processes, including group roles and member skills, is desirable to evaluate group and individual performances adequately.

Source: Adapted from *Learning Thru Discussion* by W.F. Hill, published by Sage Publications, Inc., Beverly Hills, Calif. Copyright © 1977, by permission of Sage Publications, Inc.

seem to elicit compliance but it often results in underlying resentment. Instead, change "we" statements to "I" statements. The "I" statement offers a possible solution from the speaker's point of view and allows room for others to express their beliefs about the subject.

Avoid personal put-downs.

"Your work is never on time." "You're always asking irrelevant questions." "I noticed both of your chins." "The only reason you received a raise is because you're married and I'm single." These statements almost certainly will create open and/or passive hostility because they attack the person rather than the problem. The most common response to a put-down is a counterattack. As a result, individuals become locked in an ego conflict rather than working cooperatively to solve a problem (Hawley & Hawley, 1975). Put-downs result in hostility, retreat, and withdrawal or passive hostile submission.

Accept the thoughts, feelings, beliefs, and ideas of others uncon-ditionally.

This is much easier to say than to do. In fact, it strongly tests the instructor's own value system as it relates to valuing the uniqueness of others. While acceptance does not imply agreement, it does indicate respect for beliefs and ideas that are not held personally. Without unconditional acceptance, students will not share their beliefs openly and honestly. The risks are too great.

Work toward a psychologically safe classroom climate.

The United States Constitution and Bill of Rights were written as guidelines for the relationships of one individual with another. A concern for fair treatment is at the core of each document:

- treat others fairly, even if they differ from you
- accept diversity of race and sex
- respect the individual.

Respect for diversity makes it impossible for one person to impose a belief system on another and promotes a psychologically safe classroom.

Strive to eliminate any tendency to moralize.

When individuals strive to express their thoughts and feelings, they often send messages that appear to moralize. This will stop an open discussion quickly and only students who hold similar beliefs will continue to participate.

Develop listening skills.

Listening and observing are at the core of effective discussion. In spite of the importance of these two traits to the success of a session, nursing instructors and practitioners frequently do not possess essential listening skills. Effective listening depends on the cooperation of both instructor and student. Good listeners are astute observers whose positive actions reveal unconditional acceptance and interest.

Since listening is the key to understanding, it is vital that the instructor attend to both verbal and nonverbal cues (Schulman, 1974). Competent listening assumes the mental recording of such nonverbal cues as posture (e.g., stiff or rigid, or relaxed) and accessibility (open: arms and hands loosely placed in lap; closed: arms held across chest) and such verbal cues as word choice (I think, feel, may, ought to, etc.), distance (i.e., you, they, it, we), interpretive words (cooperative, elated, normal), and voice control (voice trembles or is under smooth control).

The instructors must be able to link nonverbal and verbal cues. They interrelate in several ways:

- Repeating: A nonverbal cue may be repeated by a verbal one. For example, a gesture may be used to repeat the verbal explanation of the size of a burn area.
- Contradicting: Nonverbal cues may contradict the spoken word. For example, instructors may say they are concerned about each student's progress. However, in practice they may never be available to give review help. When there is doubt—when the verbal and nonverbal cues are contradictory—individuals will trust the latter. Actions, in reality, do speak louder than words.
- Substituting: Individuals sometimes use nonverbal cues in place of words. For example, a pat on the arm or holding the hand of a patient may be more comforting than words. A disapproving frown is an effective way to communicate disapproval.
- Complementing: Complementary nonverbal messages add to or modify verbal ones. For example, a student may respond to a question in the discussion and the tone of voice and body actions may indicate nervousness. These cues give the instructor a more accurate picture of the situation.
- Accenting: Many nonverbal cues emphasize or accent verbal ones. For example, students may place their hands on their chests to emphasize felt grief or may clench their fists to emphasize anger.
- Relating and regulating: Many nonverbal cues help individuals regulate their conversations. This helps them avoid interrupting conversations. Many parents criticize their children for interrupting when in reality the youngsters have not yet learned to link nonverbal and verbal cues to determine when it is time to participate in the conversation.

Successful leadership of a group discussion also requires the instructor to develop communication skills. In addition to the communication skills described more completely in Chapter 4 (attending behavior, paraphrasing, reflection of feeling, and summarizing content) Taba (1967) suggests these additional skills for effective discussions:

- Focusing: This enables the instructor, through skilled use of a set, to help the group focus on the specific task. A set is a brief activity that prepares students for learning. For example, for a lesson on overpopulation, the instructor may begin the class in a small closet. This brief introduction to the lesson is called a set.
- Refocusing: This often is necessary when the group has strayed from the original topic.

- Changing the focus: This is necessary when the group obviously has exhausted the topic.
- Recapping: This sort of summarizing helps students draw relationships and understand the implications of the discussion.

Developing Questioning Skills

Questioning is one of the most effective methods by which instructors can stimulate students. Effectively developed questions can focus learning and promote thoughtfulness.

Once a simple eliciting question has been made as part of the lesson in the affective domain, there will be frequent occasions when students' responses can be strengthened, expanded, or altered through the skillful use of probing questions.

Probing questions can help guide students to a more complete response. They are more likely to be needed when an attempt is made to discuss issues at the valuing level of the affective domain. This level requires students to begin to internalize their personal attitudes or beliefs. In addition to expanding and improving responses, these questions also can help increase student participation and decrease instructor talk (Bowling, n.d.).

There are five categories of probing questions: prompting, justification, clarification, extension, and redirection. Each category is analyzed next.

Prompting Questions

These are used by the instructor when the student's first response is weak, partially correct, or incorrect. The instructor follows up on these responses with a question or series of questions containing hints or clues to the desired answers. However, for the higher levels of the affective domain, there often is no precise correct or desired response. At these levels, prompting questions can be used to encourage or support a student who is reluctant to respond. The following dialogues illustrate the instructor's use of prompting to elicit a more correct response and to encourage reluctant students.

Example 1: Prompting to elicit a more correct response.

Instructor: Research studies have identified several conditions that patients believe to be necessary for humanized health care. Cindy, can you remember any of these conditions?

Cindy: Well, Mrs. Wyman said she wanted to be treated more like a person and not referred to as the "amputee in 304."

Instructor: What were her other major complaints?

Cindy: Well, she wanted some say in the decision to operate and she wanted to be treated with more empathy.

Instructor: You have just identified two conditions patients views as necessary for humanized health care—the right to exercise some control over the medical events in their lives and the need to be treated with warmth and empathy.

Example 2: Prompting to encourage a student who is reluctant to respond.

Instructor: Would you knowingly bring into the world a child with Down's syndrome?

Elizabeth: [Silence.]

Instructor: What personal or monetary costs are associated with Down's syndrome?

Elizabeth: Well, the total monetary costs are not known but they are great because individuals are affected for all their lives. The "costs" in personal suffering also are immense.

Instructor: Based on your answer, would you knowingly have a child with Down's syndrome?

Elizabeth: I don't think so, but it would be a difficult decision.

By prompting, the instructor was able to obtain an insightful response from Elizabeth. If the instructor had ignored her silence, she would have lost the opportunity to contribute.

Justification Questions

These are used to encourage students to provide a rationale for their response or to explain further why they answered as they did. Such questions help the instructor answer the following concerns: Does the student understand the answer? Do I completely understand the student's response? The following dialogue illustrates the instructor's use of justification questions:

Instructor: Will society ever have the right to mandate that a woman terminate a pregnancy?

Steven: I think so.

Instructor: Steve, can you provide some reasons for your response?

Steven: Well, it may seem unlikely now that we could enact laws requiring abortion but 30 years ago who would have believed the Supreme Court would permit abortion? The choice would be difficult but if our natural resources such as food or water became scarce people may be forced to make tough decisions.

Instructor: Steven, your response was insightful.

Again, asking a justification question, the instructor was able to elicit a more carefully thought out response from Steven. This contributed to both the quality of the discussion and to Steven's feelings of accomplishment.

Clarification Questions

These are useful when the response is inadequately organized or incomplete. The instructor then asks the student to rephrase or explain the answer. Consequently, clarification questions are used when the response is unclear or capable of being misunderstood. The following dialogue illustrates the instructor's use of clarification questions:

Instructor: After a genetic counseling session, how do you determine whether the individual understood the information?

Sara: Make sure he understands the form.

Instructor: But how can we be certain the individual understands?

Sara: Well, we can ask the person to repeat or summarize what was said, so we can check for understanding that way.

Instructor: Yes, that's good. Can we do anything else?

Sara: We can provide literature that describes the appropriate genetic counseling information. Of course, the literature must be in laymen's terms.

Instructor: Sara, you have successfully identified two good techniques for increasing understanding: (1) asking the person to repeat or summarize what was said to check for understanding and (2) providing appropriately written literature.

Extension Questions

These require a student to expand on a response by providing additional information or a more complete explanation of the answer. Extension questions help the student further consider the implications of the response and understand its relationship to other information discussed in class. The following dialogue illustrates the instructor's use of extension questions:

Instructor: How would you explain the statement, "Act always toward the other as an end, not as a means?"

Teresa: We should love individuals for themselves, not for what they can do for us.

Instructor: Would you give us an example?

Teresa: Well, my cousin, Phyllis, has Down's syndrome. Some family members believe this has been a "blessing" because it has made the family closer and it is teaching sharing and compassion to Phyllis's brother and sister. But it disturbs me because I think they are using Phyllis as a means and not an end.

Instructor: Teresa, thank you for sharing that personal example.

Redirection Questions

These are used by the instructor when the same question is asked of more than one student. Redirected questions can be used to solicit the attitudes and values of several students as they relate to a single question. This gives more students the opportunity to contribute to the discussion so their participation increases. The following dialogue illustrates the instructor's use of redirected questions:

> *Instructor:* Should genetic screening be used to identify fetuses with abnormalities for the purpose of determining whether abortion should occur?
> *Darlene:* No, I would object to any procedure that would take a human life.
> *Instructor:* Teresa, how would you respond to that question?
> *Teresa:* I believe the expense of caring for the genetically defective and the suffering of affected individuals and their families is too great not to consider abortion.

The Dynamics of Questioning for Discussions

Following are guidelines to consider when questioning (Bowling, n.d.):

Vary the technique used to encourage student participation.

For example, the instructor can address a question to the entire group. This allows all students to consider a response. Then a specific student is called on for an answer. A question can be directed to a specific student. This can encourage a shy or inattentive person to participate.

The instructor also can ask for volunteers. This allows students to participate when they believe they have an appropriate response. However, instructors should be aware of the student who monopolizes the discussion at the expense of other class members.

Reinforce Responses.

The instructor's ability to reinforce responses is crucial to the development of a good discussion. For many instructors, reinforcement is a natural part of their teaching behavior; for others, it must be consciously learned.

Four kinds of positive reinforcement can be used during discussion (Allen & Ryan, 1969):

1. Positive, direct verbal reinforcement: This occurs when the instructor immediately follows a desired response with such comments as, "I like your thinking on that issue," "Good," "Excellent," "That

shows exceptional insight,'' or other statements that indicate satisfaction with the answer.

2. Positive nonverbal reinforcement: This occurs when the instructor
immediately follows a desired response with a nonverbal message
that indicates satisfaction with the answer. Eye contact, affirmatively
nodding the head as the student speaks, moving toward the student,
or writing the response on the board are examples of nonverbal
reinforcement.

3. Qualified or partial positive reinforcement: This occurs when the
instructor reinforces part of the response. In the following, reinforcement of a partially correct answer together with another question
allow the student to give a more accurate response:

> *Instructor:* Erica, what is a common reaction of health professionals when
> working with an incurably ill patient?
> *Erica:* I think they may be apt to abandon the patient.
> *Instructor:* You're right, but what kind of abandonment takes place?
> *Erica:* Both physical and psychological abandonment are common.

4. Delayed reinforcement: This occurs when the instructor refers to a
student's previous response. In the following, the instructor reinforces both students by drawing the class's attention to Karen's
earlier contribution and praising Sandra for deducing the answer to
the original question:

> *Instructor:* What is one of the less obvious risks of placebo use?
> *Sandra:* The patient may not be helped.
> *Instructor:* Yes, that is an obvious possibility, but do you remember Karen's
> presentation on the nurse-patient relationship?
> *Sandra:* Yes, she said trust was essential. Possibly the loss of trust may be
> a risk factor in the use of a placebo.
> *Instructor:* Good deductive thinking!

Obviously, reinforcement must be appropriate to the response given.
Saying "Excellent" to an average response is ridiculous. Yet, skillfully
used, reinforcement increases student participation in the classroom.

Wait.

Many instructors have difficulty coping with silence in the classroom.
Consequently, they do not allow adequate time for formulating answers.
If students observe that an instructor rarely provides much time for thinking through a response, they will say they do not know the answer when,
in reality, if sufficient time had been allowed, they could have answered
correctly.

Rowe (1978) reported that for some instructors, wait time averages only about one second. However, if the wait time is extended, students increase their responses, more of them volunteer, slower ones join in, and instructors raise their expectations (Rowe, 1978). To increase effectiveness with wait time, instructors can:

- consciously increase wait time to five seconds
- inform students that they will have some time to formulate their answers
- ask students not to respond or volunteer during allotted wait time.

Write out some key questions before the class.

The new instructor, or the experienced one trying a new method, may find it extremely useful to plan some questions in advance.

Benefits of Discussion

A major benefit of class discussion is that it requires instructors to use questioning as an integral, constructive part of teaching. When instructors increase their skills in the use of questioning, students are encouraged to develop higher levels of thinking. Questioning requires class members to compare, contrast, consider implications, criticize, evaluate, and problem solve. It helps them to go beyond the mere repeating of facts and apply new information. Obviously, questioning should not be intimidation but rather a mutual search for knowledge. In the end, questioning is a skill that instructors can learn with planning and practice.

The discussion technique is applicable to a wide range of affective topics at all levels of nursing programs. It requires minimal physical facilities and involves all the students.

Discussion may assist in the development of new insights that precipitate fundamental attitude changes. If discussion is to do so, a great deal of planning must precede a seemingly effortless performance. Adequate instructor preparation includes (1) a thorough knowledge of the subject, (2) possession or acquisition of discussion skills, (3) a basic sensitivity to student needs, and (4) active listening skills.

Discussion also helps facilitate an atmosphere of mutual inquiry and basic trust. The most successful discussion leaders are instructors who are open, encourage student participation, and support a basic foundation of trust within the group. This supportive environment facilitates mutual inquiry and the belief that all ideas are an important contribution to the group.

Potential Weaknesses of Discussion

Effective group discussions obviously are time consuming so instructors need to make careful decisions regarding linking objectives to classroom strategies. For example, the lecture is a recommended method for cognitive objectives, discussion for affective objectives.

The discussion technique is difficult to use with large classes. A practical number is no more than 15 to 20 students. However, large groups can be broken into smaller sets if discussion leaders are available.

THE CASE STUDY METHOD

The case study method is an approach to a real or theoretical situation faced by a person, group, or organization. Learners examine all dimensions of the problem and are responsible for solving it themselves.

This method can be used by educators to develop or enhance students' capacity to deal effectively with real-life problems in a complex and changing environment (Fisher, 1978). Case studies thus are used (1) to develop skill in problem solving, (2) to provide actual opportunities for problem solving, (3) to develop analytical and decision-making capabilities, and (4) to develop human relation concepts and practical judgments.

Factors in Planning to Use Case Studies

The case study method is excellent for areas of knowledge that consider the dynamics of social, organizational, and ethical relationships. Case studies were used in the training of social workers as early as shortly after the Civil War. Later in the 19th century, the method was adopted by the Harvard Law School and, in the early 1920s, the Harvard Business School, as a result of which it is referred to as the "Harvard Case Method" (Andrews, 1956).

The following examples provide a glimpse into the unlimited range of problem areas:

- a nursing instructor faced with a low-achieving student with an IQ of 140
- a physician who refuses to fully discuss the possible side effects of a drug with patients
- a patient faced with the decision of a high-risk but life-extending major operation

- a nurse faced with an irate mother claiming her child is being treated inappropriately
- a nursing home administrator who realizes that if the nurse/patient ratio is not increased the facility will go bankrupt
- a nursing school dean faced with a no-confidence vote from the faculty because of a decision on faculty retrenchment
- a nurse torn between meeting the expectations of administration and the nursing care needs of patients
- a nurse torn between "unionism" and "professionalism."

The subjects available for case studies are limitless. Case studies present problems, dilemmas, and ethical questions, offering students an advance look at real life.

However, a case study offers only a small piece of reality; it never is possible to provide all the facts. When first introduced to case studies, students invariably ask for more facts to clarify the issues. This can be frustrating to an instructor since, as in real life, all the information desired for decision making rarely is available. The case study has no neat beginning or ending but rather presents only a small slice of reality. This is the way it is in actuality: decision-makers seldom have all the information they would like, even in this era of the so-called "information explosion."

The case study is a problem for the student to solve, so the instructor should assume the role of a learning resource team member. In that role, the instructor should be (1) knowledgeable about the subject, (2) informed as to group dynamics, (3) an astute observer of human behavior, and (4) familiar with the decision-making process.

The theoretical framework of the case study method is the discovery approach to student learning. Bruner (1961) describes discovery as the act of obtaining information for oneself rather than the originating or "discovery" of what previously was unknown to mankind. The major hypothesis of discovery learning is that categorization enhances retention and transfer of knowledge. Bruner regards this as of primary importance.

The advantages of discovery learning are that it (1) increases intellectual potency (i.e., when students acquire information by discovery, that material then is readily available for problem solving), (2) increases intrinsic motivation (i.e., the students' reward is the excitement of the discovery itself), (3) improves the technique of inquiry and helps develop problem-solving skills, and (4) increases retention and transfer of learning.

Retention and transfer of knowledge are key concepts in discovery learning. For example, they can enable students to recognize the range of anxiety symptoms in a variety of patients in a number of situations in and out of typical nursing care environments.

Procedure for the Case Study Method

The case study method involves four interdependent stages:

Stage 1: Students independently read and consider the case.

While reading the case in preparation for a discussion, the student may be asked to (1) define any technical terms or concepts presented, (2) identify major and subsidiary issues/problems, and (3) formulate a tentative analysis of the case. This last should follow a model for problem solving or case study analysis. Exhibit 3-1 presents a problem-solving model that can be used for case study analysis.

Stage 2: Students analyze and discuss the case study with others.

With a case study as a common experience, students can contribute their thoughts and react to those of others. Each helps and learns from the group. During this process they may gain new insights into their own beliefs and those of others. All sides of an issue are explored objectively in a simulation of real-world decision making.

Exhibit 3-1 Problem-Solving Model for Case Study Analysis

Setting	Clinic, home, physician's office, etc.
Statement of the Problem	Explanation of root causes Contributing factors Central/immediate problem Related problems
Assessment	Obstacles to problem solution Desired outcomes
Alternatives	Advantages/disadvantages of each alternative
Decision/Action	Rationale
Evaluation: Analysis of decision	Advantages/disadvantages Effectiveness of decision

Stage 3: Students compare their own independent analyses of the case study with those of the group.

Students may reflect on the case, the discussion, and their own decisions. They should be reminded that often there are no simple nor necessarily correct solutions nor do the studies indicate what is necessarily right or wrong. However, students do become more aware of behavioral concerns and gain vicarious experience with problem solving.

Stage 4: Students apply current experience to related and/or new ones.

As noted earlier, the case study method's theoretical framework is the discovery approach, which increases retention and transfer of students' learning. Instructors can enhance this retention and transfer potential by assisting students in applying current experience to related and/or new ones.

EXAMPLES OF CASE STUDIES

Case studies may cover an unlimited range of topics, concerns, or issues that requires judgmental decision making. They may consider (1) a single individual or a group, (2) internal relationships among departments, divisions, or groups, and (3) external relationships involving an individual's or an organization's various constituencies (Fisher, 1978).

Case studies may range from relatively simply written problems to more detailed reports that may include supporting information, the decision, and the results of the discussion. Example 1 illustrates a more detailed case. Examples 2 and 3 present shorter studies. The shorter ones obviously provide less information but offer students the opportunity to discuss and inject more of their own ideas and concerns as well as look at related issues.

Example 1: Surrogate Mothering

Identification of Subject and Sources of Information

Name: Glynnis Lynn I.
Race: Caucasian
Sex: Female
Age: 34
Education: High school graduate

Sources of information:
1. Personal observation
2. Interviews with subject
3. Interview with husband
4. Interview with siblings
5. Interview with physician

The Family History

1. Health and Physical Characteristics
The I. family consists of five members: Kenneth, the father, is 41 years old; Glynnis Lynn, the mother, 34; the sons, Philip and Robert, 11 and 12 respectively; and Leann, the daughter, 7.

All are of medium or average build. By medical standards all are in excellent health and physical condition and have not had any serious debilitating illness. All are athletically inclined and tend to excel in their chosen activities. Mrs. I. tries to be a calorie counter but enjoys food too much to permit retention of her once youthful, slender figure. She usually is just a few pounds over-weight. Mr. I. smokes but only infrequently. The entire family is considered good-looking. Their health and physical characteristics could be described in positive terms.

2. Educational Status
Both Mr. and Mrs. I. graduated from high school but neither could attend college for financial reasons. Both seem at times to resent that lack of opportunity and are determined that their children will attend college. Both boys are in middle school, Leann in elementary school. All three have above-average academic records and their names have appeared on the honor roll many times. Glynnis and Kenneth are very proud of these educational accomplishments. They have encouraged good study habits but never have pressured the children to excel.

3. Economic Status
The I. family lives in a large, older house in a quiet neighborhood. None of the neighbors are wealthy. Most families have lived there for a long time. Mr. I. works as a draftsman in a job that could best be described as "stable." Mrs. I. never has worked outside the home.

Mr. I.'s salary is adequate to meet necessities but there is no money for extras. They have a three-year-old car of medium price. They wear well-made, moderately priced, attractive cloth-ing. The home is tastefully decorated. There is a large color television set and a new stereo. Mr. and Mrs. I do not enjoy reading, so few books are evident.

4. Social Status and Adjustment

The family is active in the community, largely because of Mrs. I.'s personality. She believes friendships are important and works hard to maintain them. Mr. I. belongs to a union and attends most of its meetings. Mrs. I. is active in the Parent-Teacher Association and church and teaches Sunday school. The family life is fairly harmonious. Arguments occur but are rare. In the neighborhood the children are well known and well liked.

5. Interests and Recreation

The family likes to camp. Its yearly vacation consists of renting a camper and going to one of the state parks for a week. The members also are accomplished square dancers and attend a dance at least once a month. The entire family took square dancing lessons together. Mrs. I. is an excellent seamstress and makes many of her own and her daughter's clothes.

6. Ideology

Mr. and Mrs. I. are relatively liberal. Their basic philosophy revolves around the belief that people have the intelligence and moral responsibility to make decisions for themselves.

The Case History

Mrs. I. read an advertisement in the paper: "Couple unable to conceive, seeking surrogate mother. Financial compensation provided for loss of income and potential health risk. All medical costs and travel expenses paid. Adoptive parents accept responsibility for the child, irrespective of its state of health." Mrs. I. told her husband she would like to become a surrogate because of her sympathy for women who were unable to have children. However, she and her husband did not want any more children of their own.

Mr. I. initially was shocked when his wife approached him about the proposal. However, in the end, he accepted the idea so completely that he assisted his wife in her delivery by the Lamaze method. Both parents discussed Mrs. I.'s decision with their children.

Interpretive Questions

   1. Does impregnation of the surrogate by a married man amount to adultery?

2. What if the surrogate decides to keep the baby or have an abortion?
3. What if the adoptive parents die or are divorced before the birth?
4. What if the surrogate dies during the pregnancy because of conditions generated by it or from unrelated causes?
5. Is using a surrogate mother a valid alternative to a traditional adoption?
6. Is it fair to allow artificial insemination of the wife with the semen of a third-party donor when it is the husband who cannot have children, but not to turn to a surrogate mother when it is the wife who cannot conceive?
7. Is the surrogate being paid for the use of her body or for selling her baby?
8. Is artificial insemination morally consensual adultery?
9. Is money a hidden motive?
10. Can the surrogate mother escape emotional attachment to the child?
11. How will the surrogate and her family cope with others' hostile reactions to their decision?
12. Is surrogate motherhood unobjectionable if the goal is to provide an infertile couple with children?
13. What inferences can be made about Mrs. I.'s level of moral development? (Use Kohlberg's moral development theory as discussed in Chapter 1.)
14. What values motivated Mrs. I.'s decision?
15. Should the husband approve of the surrogate's action or walk out on or divorce her?

Finally, students are asked to justify Mrs. I.'s decision, using utilitarianism and Kantian ethics as the theoretical rationale(s).

Example 2: The Undesirable Patient

Victoria G. has been readmitted to the hospital. No one is surprised for she is well known to the emergency room staff and to most of the ward personnel. No one is happy to see her. Victoria lives in a furnished room in the Southern Hotel with several other poor, elderly individuals. Her Social Security income is enough to pay for the room and keep her drunk much of the time. Occasionally she will spend money on food but never if it means going without alcohol. She eats a daily meal at the Salvation Army.

She is being admitted with delirium tremens (DTs). Her Social Security check had been stolen so she did not have any money to keep drinking. She previously had been admitted for trauma after falling in the bathroom.

Loretta T., a young nursing student, has been visiting Victoria since her withdrawal symptoms have subsided. Victoria has come to look forward to these visits. She has told Loretta that the bottle is her best friend since all of her close relatives are dead. Her husband died a slow, painful death with lung cancer and her only son was killed in an automobile accident. Victoria says, "For me, life has no purpose. It's all right to use alcohol to 'get by.' "

Victoria appreciates the care she is getting in the hospital, especially the good food. However, she believes some members of the nursing staff treat her with disgust. She told Loretta: "I'm an alcoholic, you know, and the worst kind, a woman! They treat me like they hate me. They don't care if I live or die and neither do I. The nurses act so holy and proud, especially Mrs. O. She never even calls me by my given name. She just shouts orders and leaves as soon as possible. It's my life. I got a right to drink if I want to."

Victoria appears to have no respect for herself or her life. She merely tolerates living. She knows alcohol will kill her sooner or later and she doesn't care.

Loretta also has observed Nurse O.'s subtle hostile interactions with Victoria. Loretta's mother had struggled with alcoholism until her early death so Loretta has witnessed the power of alcohol addiction and has no illusions that she could convince Victoria to stop drinking. However, she is upset by Nurse O.'s attitude. Loretta shares her concerns with Janet L., a staff nurse. Mrs. L. listens, then says: "Loretta, this is your first clinical experience. I understand your feelings. Maybe you're right that Mrs. G. is not being treated with respect. But remember there are a lot of patients here that need our time and there is much you do not know. Besides, with all the talk about the hospital merger, the first rule around here is survival. Wait before you do anything you'll be sorry for later."

The next day Loretta is visiting with Victoria when Nurse O. enters the room with a syringe on a tray. "You," she says, "turn over, it's time for your shot." Victoria protests but Nurse O. insists, gives the injection, and leaves immediately. Victoria overhears her outside the room telling another staff member that she is "Looney as a hoot owl because of the brain damage caused by the alcohol abuse. If she gives me any grief and continues to be uncooperative, I'll tell her doctor."

Victoria is humiliated, embarrassed, and angry. She quietly vows to leave the hospital and never return.

Now Loretta is more distressed than ever. Is there a "double standard" for caring? Aren't all patients valued as unique individuals? Can't a better relationship be developed between Victoria and Nurse O.? What can Loretta do? To whom can she turn for support? At what point can she relinquish responsibility for further action?

Critical reasoning or problem-solving models are recommended for analysis of the case study. Exhibit 3-2 illustrates the application of the problem-solving model previously presented in an actual case.

Example 3: The Case of the Siamese Twins

Parents of Siamese twins born in Danville, Ill., had ordered that they not be fed. The twins were joined at the waist with a

---

Exhibit 3-2 Application of Problem-Solving Model to a Case Study

Setting	Hospital
Statement of the Problem	Relate the behavior of Loretta T., Mrs. O., and Janet L. to Kohlberg's stages of moral development.
	What is the immediate problem? What are the related problems? What are the contributing factors to the problem?
Assessment	Obstacles to problem solving: Why are the feelings toward Victoria so strong? Why is it difficult for Mrs. O. to act with respect toward Victoria? Why is Loretta able to feel and express more compassion than the other members of the staff? What are the desired outcomes?
Alternatives	What alternatives are available to Loretta? Describe the advantages and disadvantages of each.
Decision/Action	Rationale
Evaluation: Analysis of the decision	Advantages/disadvantages Effectiveness of the decision

common pelvis and bowel. A third, defective leg protruded from one side. The parents and the physician were charged with attempted murder. (*The Herald-Leader,* 1981).

Interpretive Questions

1. What inferences can be drawn about the parents' values?
2. What inferences can be made about the parents' level of moral development? (Use Kohlberg's [1975] moral development theory.)
3. What are the possible alternatives, the decision, and its implications? (Use the problem-solving model for case study analysis.)

Additional nursing dilemma case studies are included in Appendix 3-A.

Benefits of Case Studies

The case study approach can simulate reality. It offers students an opportunity to experience real-life issues and problems vicariously. This experience is relatively failure free as students share potential solutions, applying a rational   approach to decision making.

This approach offers a variety of problem-solving experiences that are excellent for many educational objectives. It encourages students to analyze entire chains of causal events and their contributing factors, anticipate consequences, discuss possible long-term and short-term outcomes, and identify the potential implications of various decisions.

The method can provide the functional link between theory and practice, between the classroom and the real world. It offers students the opportunity to transfer concepts and principles to sound decision making. Obviously the method does not provide necessarily correct solutions to the problems being studied nor does it indicate what is correct or incorrect. However, it does provoke critical thinking and helps students realize that there are no magic solutions (Fisher, 1978).

The case study method can be fun. Since it considers material that is current, approximates reality, and involves students in an empathetic, active way, it can be enjoyable. It also promotes purposeful, unified learning experiences that can be shared by the students and the instructor.

Limitations of the Case Study

The limitations of the case study discussed here are not those of the method itself but rather in how it is used.

The instructor may have difficulty writing and/or developing good case study material. However, studies may be prepared by colleagues in the field, alumni of the program, and students as part of the learning experience. Obviously first drafts will need to be edited carefully, precautions should be taken to conceal actual identities of people and/or places, and the case material must be congruent with course objectives.

Students may lack sufficient experience to assess the case study adequately. Some study material may be so complex that students do not have the necessary knowledge and/or experiences to analyze the problem adequately. Obviously the instructor must choose case studies that are appropriate to the levels of the educational objectives.

ROLE PLAYING

Role playing is an action technique in which two or more people first act out a realistic problem by drawing on information they are given, then follow up with a group discussion of the experience.

The purposes of role playing are varied. For classroom teaching it often is used to (1) create insight into the attitudes and motives of others, (2) create an awareness of how each student affects others, and (3) develop skills in selected interpersonal processes.

For the first two purposes, the situational outcome is secondary to the students' ability to perceive the feelings, attitudes, and intentions inherent in the characters played.

For the third use, that of developing interpersonal skills (such as the affective ones of expressing empathy, displaying positive regard, reducing threat, and developing trust) and communication skills (e.g., attending behavior, paraphrasing, reflecting feelings, and summarizing content) the situational context is of primary importance. The success of the role playing will depend on the students' ability to apply these interpersonal skills (King, 1979).

Immediately following the role playing, the process is analyzed. For instructors to serve most effectively as discussion leaders, they need skills in observation, analysis, and group dynamics. The use of discussion is a critical component of this teaching technique.

Role playing promotes the students' intellectual, emotional, and physical involvement; stimulates creativity; and maintains interest. Role playing may be (1) open-ended (players are given only a problem and a role), (2) structured (greater detail is provided about the problems and roles), or (3) directed (a word-for-word script is provided). As noted earlier, role playing is very effective for affective learning.

Factors in Planning to Use Role Playing

While role playing is only a simulation of real experience, students do become highly emotionally involved in the activity. As a result the instructor must be extremely sensitive to both the topic and its possible effect on specific students. For example, one whose mother has just died of lung cancer may find it difficult to role-play with a lung cancer patient.

As noted, instructors should be skilled in observation, analysis, group dynamics, and the use of discussion as a technique. Both Piaget (1948) and Kohlberg (1975) suggest that talk can be one of the significant influences in changing the cognitive functioning and behavior of the young. In addition to the instructors' special skills of observation and the use of discussion there also must be no hint of authority or special status and no suggestion of what solution the student should follow. In other words, talk between students and the instructor must be conducted as if between peers to affect behavior.

Role playing is a skill, therefore it must be practiced to be learned. It is a good classroom method for learning human interaction techniques. It provides the observers with a complex, complete repertoire of skills to imitate. While role playing, students think, feel, and act simultaneously as they are completely involved in the situation. As a result, cognition, affect, and psychomotor skills are being demonstrated simultaneously. Role playing resembles life more closely than do many other teaching methodologies.

Social imitation learning, thought to represent the main avenue through which personality characteristics are acquired, can be enhanced by role playing. Much human learning is a function of observing the behavior of others (Bandura & Walters, 1963). Furthermore, those experts believe that people learn to imitate through being reinforced for so doing, and that continued reinforcement maintains imitative behavior. Consequently, observational behavior may be fundamental to acquiring new behaviors or to modify old ones.

Procedure for Conducting a Role-Playing Activity

Educators who have discussed various phases in role playing (Liveright, 1951; Bavelas, 1977) suggest anywhere from three to 14 steps in the activity. However, this discussion offers only four.

Phase 1 involves preparation of the participants and observers. The instructor should begin each role-playing activity by providing as much information as possible. This may include the following:

- A brief description of the role-playing incident.
  Tonia was bathing a small boy with cystic fibrosis. He had been admitted in critical condition, with serious pulmonary involvement. However, he was doing much better and was receiving respiratory therapy. There was a huge teddy bear in his bed that also was wearing an oxygen mask. Tonia asked the boy how the teddy bear was feeling. He responded, "He's dying."
- A description of roles to be assumed during the role play.
  Patient's role: The patient is Michael Abrams, 9 years old. You love to play arcade games, especially Moon Cresta at Galaxie of Games. You collect matchbox cars and baseball cards. You enjoy drawing and are afraid that you are dying. You are hospitalized frequently.
  Nurse's role: The nurse is Tonia Armstrong, 20 years old. You have a healthy 11-year-old brother. You are a third-year nursing student and have spent the previous three summers working in a nursing home. You enjoy working in pediatrics. Your grandfather has died recently. You are frustrated because you have an opportunity to discuss dying with Michael but are finding it difficult. At first you are silent, then you respond to Michael by saying, ". . ."
- A list of objectives for the role-playing exercises.
  Cognitive objectives: The student will be able to describe the stages of death and dying. The student will be able to describe the etiology, symptomatology, diagnostic procedures, and treatment for cystic fibrosis.
  Affective objectives: The student will be able to listen to patients expressing feelings about death. The student will be able to express warmth and empathy.
  (One role-playing activity may accomplish objectives in more than one learning domain simultaneously.)

Phase 2 calls for enactment of the role-playing incident. Interaction among group members through role playing is the core of this phase. Before starting this phase, the instructor must assign roles to appropriate students and prepare the physical environment.

Phase 3, analysis and discussion, is a critical component of the sequence. As mentioned earlier, the instructor should be able to use group discussion to facilitate meeting the objectives. The analysis and discussion help prepare for future role playing or more traditional learning strategies.

The instructor's ability to facilitate discussion is crucial to this phase. It should be made clear to the group members that the goal is not to criticize other role players but rather to participate in a nonthreatening environment, experiment with new behaviors, become more sensitive to the feelings and concern of others, and maintain an unconditionally accepting atmosphere. The effective use of questioning skills will make this phase more productive.

This phase also may include an informal critique or evaluation. The class may discuss the positive aspects of the session and recommend areas where improvement might be made. For example, the instructor might encourage the use of a teacher-made rating scale to assess communication, counseling, or interviewing skills.

Students directly involved in the role playing may want to talk over their feelings and reactions to the activity individually with the instructor before it is discussed with the entire class.

Phase 4, summarization and closure, provides that the instructor, a student, or the entire class may recapitulate the role-playing incident, extracting some general principles that were related to the experience in the process.

Closure links new knowledge to previous information and serves as a cognitive link to future learning. Closure can assist students in drawing relationships and forming an organization for transfer. It goes beyond merely summarizing what has occurred.

Allen and Ryan (1969) offer three useful approaches to assisting students toward closure; they also help the instructor determine whether closure has been achieved:

1. Review and summary. During the discussion phase of the role-playing activity students often stray from the topic and bring up only tangential points. It is important for the instructor to listen to what has been said, then abstract and summarize the main ideas and relate them to the activity.

2. Application of current experiences to related ones. For example, after Tonia's experiences with Michael are discussed, the group can turn to the care of previous patients with similar problems. This process can assist the students in extracting generalizations from specifics.

3. Extension of current learning to new situations. This assists students in transferring information from one situation to another. For example, after analyzing Tonia's experiences with Michael, the students can discuss the care of future patients with similar concerns. This will help them understand that any patient with a terminal illness may have the same concerns as Michael.

The use of closure has several benefits: It can provide students with a feeling of achievement and, equally important, it can facilitate the transfer of learning.

To summarize, Johnson (1965) separates instructional closure from cognitive closure. Instructional closure is accomplished when the instructor has described the link between past knowledge and new knowledge. By contrast, cognitive closure has been achieved when the students can link old and new information.

EXAMPLES OF ROLE-PLAYING EXERCISES

This section provides examples of three types of role-playing exercises: (1) the open-ended, (2) the structured, and (3) the directed. Each example includes directions, evaluations (if appropriate), the setting, roles, and objectives. Each is designed to stimulate the instructor.

The variation and potential of topics for role-playing activities are limitless. Ideas can be generated from students, from past experiences, and from other faculty members. For example, if the instructor would like to use directed role-playing exercises, scripts can be written from appropriate fiction or nonfiction books.

Role playing can be an effective teaching strategy. The participants strive to assume the attitudes, values, and feelings that would represent those of the individuals involved in the situation. In so doing, they find themselves in face-to-face confrontation with a real person with real feelings.

Example 1: Open-Ended Role-Playing Exercise

Directions:

1. Select two participants to do the role playing.
2. Determine the appropriate amount of time for the role playing.
3. Determine who will lead the discussion and assessment that will follow.
4. Give specific directions to the nurse (i.e., to counsel the mother regarding her concerns for her daughter, Annie, her husband, and herself).
5. Read The Setting (infra) to all the observers.

Evaluation

After completion of the role-playing exercise, the students complete the evaluation form provided (Exhibit 3-3). The group leader and the observers then discuss the extent to which the player

Exhibit 3-3 Role-Playing Evaluation Form

Were the following phases for implementing the role-playing activity accomplished:			
			Comments
1. Phase 1. The instructor began the role-playing activity by providing:			
a. A brief description of the role-playing incident.	Yes	No	
b. A description of the roles to be assumed during the role play.	Yes	No	
c. A list of objectives for the exercise.	Yes	No	
2. Phase 2. Enactment of the role-playing incident.	Yes	No	
3. Phase 3. Analysis and discussion.	Yes	No	
4. Phase 4. Summarization and closure.	Yes	No	
How would you rate the overall effectiveness of the lesson?			
1 = not effective			
2 = somewhat effective			
3 = effective			
4 = very effective			
COMMENTS:			

who assumed the role of the nurse adequately exhibited the affective skills of expressing empathy (demonstrated positive regard and developed trust) and the communication skills of (1) attending behavior, (2) paraphrasing, (3) reflecting feeling, and (4) summarizing content (Table 3-2). Finally the person who played the nurse should be prepared to listen to a critique of the interview with the person who played the mother. Note that Table 3-2 could also be used to assess communication skills between students and instructors.

The Setting (read to all observers)

Annie H. is a 3-year-old child with a congenital heart defect; she is often hospitalized. During her present hospital stay her mother is extremely worried.

Roles

The mother sits with her legs tightly crossed and her hands clasped in her lap. Her facial expression is sad yet anxious. She looks at the nurse, and says in a concerned voice: "I just don't know what to do. I'm afraid to hold Annie. I'm afraid she may stop

Table 3-2 Scale for Rating Communication Skills

Attending Behavior	Paraphrasing	Reflecting Feeling	Summarizing Content
Level 1 Listener responds in a distant, unrelated manner; verbal and nonverbal responses indicate little attention to patient's behavior. Listener persistently shifts position and moves about.	**Level 1** Listener rarely rewords or repeats important statements.	**Level 1** Listener rarely reflects patient's feelings accurately.	**Level 1** Listener does not attempt to summarize ideas and feelings expressed during interview.
Level 2 Listener communicates to patient that listener is interested in patient's responses. Listener maintains appropriate posture most of the time.	**Level 2** Listener usually rewords or repeats important statements.	**Level 2** Listener usually reflects patient's feelings accurately.	**Level 2** Listener summarizes most of ideas and feelings expressed during interview.
Level 3 Listener shows intense interest in patient's verbal and nonverbal behavior. Listener persistently maintains appropriate posture.	**Level 3** Listener consistently rewords and repeats all important statements.	**Level 3** Listener consistently and accurately reflects patient's feelings by making them known in fresh words.	**Level 3** Listener summarizes totality of ideas and feelings expressed during interview.

breathing, afraid to feed her, afraid she may choke. My husband is angry because all I do is worry. I'm not even interested in sex anymore. Is Annie going to be all right?''

The student assuming the role of the nurse has complete freedom to develop this role.

Objectives

- Cognitive: Contrast the adaptive needs of a parent whose child has an acute illness with those of one whose child has a chronic illness.
- Affective: Apply the communication skills of attending behavior, paraphrasing, reflecting feeling, and summarizing content.

Example 2: Structured Role-Playing Exercise

Directions:

1. Select three participants to do the role playing and give each a specific role.
2. Determine the appropriate amount of time for the role playing.
3. Determine who will lead the discussion and assessment that will follow.
4. Read The Setting (infra) to all the observers.

Evaluation

After completion of the role-playing exercise, the students complete the communication skills evaluation form provided (Exhibit 3-4). The group leader and the observers then discuss the extent to which the player who assumed the role of the nurse adequately exhibited communication skills in addition to knowledge of the genetic disease. Finally, the person who played the nurse should be prepared to listen to a critique of the performance with the individuals who played the patient and the spouse.

The Setting (read to all observers)

A 43-year-old executive has polycystic kidney disease—in his case, a genetic disorder. He must have hemodialysis. Victims of the disease may live as long as ten years after symptoms appear if they can obtain dialysis or a kidney transplant. However, many

Exhibit 3-4 Score Sheet for Communication Skills

Directions:
Place check under *one* of the levels for *each* characteristic. The Communication Level equals the level of the check under each category divided by 4 (the total number of categories). This is the average level for all characteristics.

Example:　Attending behavior　　Level 3
　　　　　Paraphrasing　　　　　Level 1
　　　　　Reflecting feeling　　　Level 2
　　　　　Summarizing Content　Level 2
　　　　　　　　　　Total　　= 8
　　　　　Divided by 4 = 2　(Level 2)

	Levels		
	1	2*	3
Attending behavior			
Paraphrasing	1	2	3
Reflecting feeling	1	2	3
Summarizing content	1	2	3

*Minimum communication level.

die a few years after the symptoms appear. The patient has two teen-age daughters. He and his wife both know the disease is genetic and insist the daughters not be told. They fear the information might frighten them unnecessarily, inhibit their social life, and leave them feeling hopeless about their future.

Roles

David B. is an executive of a local newspaper. He believes that his daughters should not be told about the genetic link in his kidney disease. He is hopeful that dialysis will keep him alive until his daughters are grown and self-supporting. He is reluctant to discuss this decision with nursing personnel.

Sara B., 39 years old, has been a full-time homemaker for 13 years and has just returned to college to complete a master's degree in social work. She has been overly protective of her daughters. She seems more willing than her husband to tell them that his disease is genetic.

Robin K. is a 33-year-old registered nurse. She has worked full time for ten years and has been active in the women's rights movement. She believes the family should share all available medical information. She must talk with Mr. and Mrs. B. about their decision.

Objectives

- Cognitive: Describe the etiology, symptomatology, treatment modalities, and complications of polycystic kidney disease.
- Affective: Explore inferences about the personal value systems of David B., Sara B., and Robin K.

Example 3: Directed Role-Playing Exercise

Directions:

1. Select four participants to do the role playing and give each a specific role.
2. Determine who will lead the discussion and assessment that will follow.
3. Read The Setting (infra) to all the observers.

Evaluation

There is no evaluation form for this exercise since the role play is completely scripted. The primary purpose is to stimulate discussion concerning the importance of patient education and communication in the nursing process. This exercise may be used as a set induction. Set inductions provide a cognitive bridge to what will follow in the instructional sequence. They are particularly appropriate (1) at the beginning of a class, (2) before classroom discussion, or (3) preceding a new clinical experience.

The Setting (read to all observers)

Belinda is a 21-year-old white student-teacher. She is married to a medical student. She has complained of headaches since she was in the fourth grade. She has returned from classes with a raging headache. Her husband found her crouched in a corner of the bed, with the lights out. He promptly took her to the hospital emergency room. Her subsequent experiences are presented in Exhibit 3-5 (Daniel, 1980).

Exhibit 3-5 Directed Role-Playing Exercise

Nurse:	Hey, how are you feeling? Sorry we have to check on you so early. Are you O.K.?
Belinda:	My headache is still bad and I've had dry heaves, nausea, and dizziness. (Patient begins to hyperventilate.)
Nurse:	Has this ever happened to you before?
Belinda:	(Sarcastically) Oh, sure! I do it all the time. (Patient is given oxygen and her cramped arms and feet are massaged. She groans in pain.)
Nurse:	Can you open your eyes for me? Try to relax. You'll be fine. You have been scheduled for an emergency brain scan.
Belinda:	This must be some kind of joke.
Nuclear Medicine Technician:	Are you Belinda?
Belinda:	(Sarcastically) No, I'm Athena in disguise.
Nuclear Medicine Technician:	O.K., we're ready for you. Here, drink this and finish it all.
Belinda:	(Thinking: She nearly got hit by projectile vomiting. Nothing must be seriously wrong or they wouldn't be taking so long. No big deal.)
Nuclear Medicine Technician:	O.K., we're ready for you. Lie on the table and we will start the scan in about 30 minutes. This will sting a little.
Belinda:	(Thinking: That shot hurt way inside me. I thought my head would explode.)
Nuclear Medicine Technician:	O.K., let me help you down. Sit in the chair by the drum. Lay your head against this surface and hold it there. Good!
Belinda:	(Thinking: This is becoming a Gothic nightmare. My head is strapped to the high drum so tightly I can't move. The drone of those computers in this little room is numbing my poor, aching head. I nearly collapsed to the floor when he unstrapped me.)
Nuclear Medicine Technician:	Now turn your head to the right.
Belinda:	(Thinking: This could assure anyone of a raging headache, strapping and unstrapping my head to the hum of the printout results. [Later] It was lunchtime when I was returned to the floor.)
Nurse:	Where's Belinda? We need her signature on this. Hope she hasn't eaten anything yet. We have to prep her. (Belinda appears from the bathroom.) Do you know what this procedure is, hon?
Belinda:	(Slowly shakes her head.) I think I'll take a rain check on this one.
Nurse:	You're a little scared aren't you?
Radiology Technician:	I have to give you a shot. It will sting a little but it will relax you.
Belinda:	I've heard that one before.
Nurse:	She's going to have a general, isn't she?
Radiology Technician:	No. And they didn't even prep her for the angiogram.
Belinda:	(Thinking: Masked, gloved, and distant. They peered at me as I was immodestly soaped and shaved for the femoral puncture.)
Radiology Technician:	Hon, when they inject the dye through the catheter you'll feel a hot flush but lie still so we can shoot the film.
Belinda:	(Thinking: That catheter stung when it entered but I didn't feel it once it was inside.)
Radiology Technician:	Can you get into the right carotid? Hon, we have to strap your head and chin down so you won't move while we take the pictures.

Exhibit 3-5 continued

Belinda: (Thinking: It felt as though every vessel in my head exploded. I thought my eyes were going to pop out. I tried to scream to someone this was a terrible mistake.)

Radiology Technician: Let's pull out and do the other side.

Belinda: (Thinking: Surely, not again. There has never in my life been a worse nightmare. I wonder if any one of those people in green has gone through this personally. I was scared and there was nothing to help my pain.)

Radiology Technician: How ya doing, hon? Hold real still now?

Belinda: (Thinking: She didn't read my face, and my head blew apart again. I felt like blood was covering my brain. Those people in green got all blurry and I didn't care.)

Nurse: My God! Her hands and feet are like ice! Hey! You are breathing too fast. Slow down! She's too alert for having all that Valium. This shouldn't be happening. Those splotches weren't there a minute ago! Give me some benadryl! She's having a reaction!

Belinda: (Thinking: My head's still bolted to the table and they jab a needle in my shoulder.)

Radiology Technician: Is she all right now? We need to do a vertebral. Just one more time, hon, hold still.

Belinda: (Thinking: This time the hemorrhaging and ricocheting didn't even bother me. I'm too woozy. Then, they peeled off the tape.)

Radiology Technician: Go find someone to take her back to the floor. I'm ready for some lunch.

Belinda: (Thinking: I was beginning to wish I'd never said I'd had a headache. My lunch had gotten cold so they took it away.)

Source: Adapted from *Any Other Song: A Plea for Holistic Communications* by E.L. Daniel, published by the Robert J. Brady Company, Bowie, Md. Copyright ©, 1980, by permission of the Robert J. Brady Company.

Roles

Belinda has had a headache for four days, followed by dry heaves, nausea, and dizziness, all of which have persisted. She has also had an associated personality change to listlessness and apathy. The headache is bifrontal and bitemporal. Belinda is afebrile but she does complain of photophobia. She is alert, oriented, and cooperative, with normal speech, except for apathy. She has a well-healed laminectomy midline incision with chronic low back pain.

The nurse is a 29-year-old white female, married, with one 9-year-old child. She has worked full time for eight years and had considerable experience with neurosurgery patients. She has a reputation of being somewhat gruff but extremely efficient. However, she sometimes intimidates new graduates.

The nuclear medicine technician is a 32-year-old white male. He graduated from college with a degree in biology but found problems getting a job. He finally was hired in the nuclear medicine department and received on-the-job training.

The radiology technician is a 40-year-old white female. Graduated 20 years ago from a hospital-based radiologic technology program, she has three children 17, 15, and 9. She is seen by her peers as a skilled technician. However, she does not believe strongly in patient education. She has been heard to say, "The less they know, the less they worry."

Objectives:

- Cognitive: Develop a functional nursing care plan that includes patient education.
- Affective: Apply the communication skills of attending behavior, paraphrasing, reflecting feeling, and summarizing content.

Benefits of Role Playing

The emphasis is on personal concerns and personal behaviors. Through the use of role-playing incidents generated by the students, the instructor can assist in providing education directly related to their needs. For example, during a pediatric rotation the student nurse may see an infant go into anaphylactic shock after the injection of bicillin. The nurse may want to discuss feelings caused by the incident. A role-playing activity may be a way for the individual to express feelings that otherwise might be repressed. The importance of relevant personal concerns cannot be overestimated.

Active student participation is provided and the artificial separation between thoughts, words, and actions is reduced. Active participation allows the students to analyze, explore, experiment, and test new situations in a relatively risk-free environment. As a result, they can make mistakes, observe others, and try out alternative responses.

> *When I hear it, I forget.*
> *When I see it, I remember.*
> *When I do it, I know.*
> Author Unknown

Role playing can help in increasing social sensitivity (Clore & Jeffery, 1971; Stivers, Buchan, Dettloff, & Orlich, 1972). By assuming roles of others and discussing personal feelings that result, students can change their personal attitudes and increase their awareness of the feelings of others.

During discussions following role playing, students also are provided information about the feelings and beliefs of others that are rarely aired. As they become sensitive to the impact of their behavior on others they are more able to change that conduct. Feedback helps students identify areas about themselves that are open to others but closed to themselves.

Observers can help (1) identify assumptions implied by the behavior, (2) assess the impact of the conduct, and (3) identify patterns that may be a source of friction. This information can increase the sensitivity regarding the thoughts and feelings of others, improve self-understanding, and prepare the students to change their behavior.

Role playing may prepare students to change their behavior. While a completely satisfactory theory to explain the value of role playing in changing behavior has not been developed, Moreno (1953) has explored the subject. For Moreno (1953) one of the critical factors in role playing that encourages behavior change is a reduction of inhibitions. Fear of ridicule, punishment, and disapproval encourages inhibitions. In contrast, a role-playing environment that provides unconditional acceptance makes exploration of attitudes, values, and beliefs possible. Consequences of new behavior can be tested in an understanding environment. Practice can help stabilize the new behavior, allowing it to become a part of real life.

Limitation of Role Playing

It may not be suited to all teachers or all students. Some instructors may be unwilling to experiment for several reasons: (1) it may be difficult for them to deal with the fact that there is no way to predict how the role play will develop and (2) role playing often deals with controversial topics and emotional issues that may be uncomfortable for some instructors. Students also may be timid and hesitate to become involved.

SIMULATION GAMING

Simulation is a representation of a real event in a reduced and compressed form that is dynamic, safe, and efficient (Rockler, 1978). A game is a contest between two or more players that has rules, goals, constraints on what can be done, and consequences for participants' behavior. There are many variations (i.e., sometimes player A can win only if player B loses, or everyone wins, or everyone loses).

The simulation game combines the elements of a simulation and a game. It can assume several variations. It can be a card game, a role-playing sequence, a board game, or a board game that integrates role playing. In nursing education, simulation gaming can be viewed as a dynamic teaching method that recreates elements of the actual nurse-patient relationship or other professional linkages (Clark, 1976). Since elements of a simulated game are patterned to represent aspects of reality, they are useful to (1) involve students actively, (2) present opportunities for creative behavior, (3) offer unique opportunities for success and recognition among peers, (4) give the teacher an opportunity to observe students in a more lifelike environment where various forms of talent and behavior may be identified, and (5) provide relevant and enjoyable educational experiences (Maley, 1978).

Simulation games also can be used to (1) help students develop strategies for living and working, (2) assist in the development of attitudes, (3) provide insight into human relations problems, (4) demonstrate the idea of cause and effect, and (5) illustrate the dynamics of problem-oriented tasks.

Nearly any game contains many essential elements of real life. A social simulation game has the power to magnify one central component of social interaction, excluding all else, and thus focuses a heightened meaning on the incident. For nursing students, simulation games can serve as an introduction to clinical life with its corresponding rules, roles, and conflicts.

Another special link between games and life is the development in psychiatry that describes an emphasis on the often destructive behavior adults use toward others. For example, in *Games People Play,* Eric Berne (1964) describes the "games" people engage in as part of everyday life such as games of subtle intimidation. Consequently, games in all forms have great potential for educators and have just as much potential for teaching as a chapter in a textbook or a lecture.

The defense of games culminates in the work of John Dewey (1928), who examines their functions for society in general and the educational system in particular. Dewey views play as a positive function in itself; he even assigns a positive moral value to games. He believes that play and games not only fill a basic human need for make-believe activity but also provide fresh and deeper meanings to everyday occurrences.

The role-playing aspect of games contributes to a socialization function by allowing players to experience a variety of roles. The role-playing characteristic in many social simulation games is viewed as an outgrowth of the technique of psychodrama developed in the 1930s by Moreno. In Moreno's research with delinquent girls, he concluded that they did not have the necessary experiences to prepare them for life outside of institutions. Starting with simple simulated situations in which subjects acted out their personal problems, role-playing sessions were extended in scope and complexity (Moreno, 1953). Similarly, many social simulation games resemble psychodrama in that players tend to get deeply involved in their game roles.

The available evidence seems to justify a general claim that simulation games are not just a reprive from "real" learning but may have a direct impact, so that even brief playing sessions include measurable effects (Boocock & Schild, 1981).

Factors in Planning to Use Simulation Games

While the playing of games is fun, it also is serious business (Duke, 1974). Games can lead to improved opportunity for socialization. Moore and Anderson (1960), discussing the role of games as a socializing technique, argue that individuals must learn to deal effectively with problems caused by the environment. These problems often involve human interaction. These authors suggest that individuals can learn to solve such problems by playing simulation games. To learn how to participate in activity A (where failure may result in serious consequences), instructors develop activity A^1 (a simulation). Activity A^1 lacks serious consequences; however, it is enough like activity A to provide genuine practice. Activity A^1 is a serious "game" that helps prepare students to interact in the natural and social world.

Simulation games should not be used to present theoretical learning for the first time or to replace it but rather to complement it. Theories, ideologies, and/or hypotheses should be presented first; simulations and games then can be used to test them, provide direct experience, and expand information presented in more traditional lecture and/or seminar presentations.

Simulation games are an outgrowth of sociological and psychological research. Research has provided insights into the operations of political, social, and economic systems, producing a clearer, more valid and reliable base upon which to plan and develop simulated games. For example, the research in decision making provides the conceptual framework for developing games that illustrate the differences in morale and productivity that are related to leadership style—i.e., autocratic, democratic, or laissez faire (Bernstein, 1977).

Simulation games require a redefinition of the academic environment. An open, unstructured learning environment is essential for successful simulation activities. As a result the teacher/student relationship must be restructured because most of the interaction in games is student/student. Students become responsible to their peers rather than to the instructor for their actions. The instructor assumes the role of facilitator. The role is changed from a didactic one to a more heuristic one (i.e., a method that encourages students to discover for themselves). Students learn that their actions/decisions have implications for both themselves and others. These implications are likely to be both affective and cognitive.

In some simulation games, students can teach their peers, further freeing the instructor to evaluate and individualize learning (Clark, 1976).

Procedure for Simulation Gaming in the Classroom

The initial step is to determine the objectives sought to be achieved. It should be remembered that the simulation game is an appropriate learning method only if it relates directly to a predetermined objective (Rockler, 1978).

The instructor then selects a game or designs one. Obviously, choosing a game assumes a knowledge of what is available. A selected list of simulation activities appears in Appendix 3-B. Guidelines for selecting a simulation game should consider learning objectives, relationship to curriculum, playability, and practicality (Clark, 1976):

- Learning Objectives: There should be congruity between the learning objectives and the game structure. The game experience should relate to the real clinical world.
- Relationship to the Curriculum: The instructor should ask: Where in the curriculum can a simulation game be used most effectively to reinforce other learning experiences? Is there a theoretical base in the game that reinforces a curriculum goal?
- Playability: A simulation game may seem appropriate but when played it may be fraught with unknowns and rule gaps. For example, procedural rules describing the general order in which play proceeds may be missing. Furthermore, specific assumptions about the goals of the game may be unknown. Two key questions are: Does the game include an explanation of how it was developed? Does it include information that describes how nursing students have learned from the game?
- Practicality: Several variables should be considered when considering practicality: cost (including how many games are needed for the entire class to play at the same time), time required, space needed, how many students can play at the same time, and how easily the game can be obtained.

The simulation game then is introduced to the students. This should include a complete discussion of the rules and instructions for playing. The instructor should be careful not to offer solutions or strategies.

The next step: Play the game. The role of the instructor is crucial during the simulation game. The teacher should observe and serve as a resource person with minimal involvement but should not play unless there is a stated role such as moderator described in the instructions. Some instructors may have difficulty assuming a more facilitative role. However, actions such as lecturing, describing outcomes in advance, or suggesting courses of action will seriously limit the success of the method.

Playing games is noisy so the instructor should be prepared for a change in the nature of the classroom. To the outside observer the students' behavior may seem disruptive and without purpose; however, that noisy, active, participative learning is replacing traditional passive education.

Finally, the instructor should conduct a debriefing session, focusing on the activity that took place, analyzing what happened, and attempting to generalize to other experiences. The questioning skills presented in the discussion method of this chapter can be used during the debriefing session.

After the debriefing, the instructor can provide a sense of closure by introducing no new materials, summarizing major points, and relating the simulation game to the original objective.

While evaluation of the activity is important, it should not be done during the debriefing. The students' perceptions of the effectiveness of the experiences can be given at the end of the semester when the entire course is being evaluated.

An example of a large simulation game that is relevant to nursing is *The Kidney Machine Problem* (Phillips, 1974) that appears as Appendix 3-C.

Designing a Simulation Game

Instructors who are considering designing their simulation games can find it often is a difficult process as the many poorly designed games attest. As a result, the method is criticized when in fact it is the game, not the method, that is flawed.

Rockler (1978) recommends not attempting to design a game until the instructor has had considerable experience playing those developed by others. Some of the process of designing is based on imitation. Therefore, instructors should:

- become familiar with what exists
- determine what objectives are to be achieved

- develop a cognitive map (Duke, 1974) (i.e., a mental picture of how the simulation game is arranged, how it proceeds, and what equipment is necessary)
- develop a working model of the cognitive map (a flow chart works well)
- begin actual construction of the simulation game, working back and forth refining both the flow chart and the game structure.

Designing a simulation game also includes (1) writing a scenario specifying the parameters of the activity, (2) focusing on what to omit as well as what to include, (3) devising a way for ending the game, (4) developing a debriefing guide, and (5) specifying the rules by which the game will be played. For developing a social simulation game, the following types of rules are necessary (Boocock & Schild, 1981):

Procedural Rules

Procedural rules describe how the game is to be played. In a social simulation game, the procedural rules should follow the natural order of activities in the situation being studied. For example, in a game related to family functioning, a set of procedural rules would be necessary to help resolve family conflict.

This sequence includes assumptions about family functioning.

A procedural subtype found in many games is called the mediation rule. This specifies how an impasse in play is resolved or a conflict resolved. For example, mediation rules are necessary in the *Community Response* game when two players attempt to operate the same agency or in the *Economic System Game* when workers and employer cannot agree on a wage.

Behavior Constraint Rules

These correspond to the role obligations found in real life and specify what the player must do and cannot do. They describe the role specifications for each player.

Goal Achievement Rule

This rule specifies the goal to be achieved for each type of player. Obviously the goals must correspond to those appropriate in real life and be socially acceptable.

Environmental Response Rules

These specify how the environment would behave if it actually were present as part of the game. In social simulation games, these rules are important because they provide the probable response of significant parts of the environment that are not incorporated into the game.

Police Rules

These state the consequences for breaking the rules and help serve as a referee.

Benefits of Simulation Gaming

Simulation gaming contributes to the building of students' self-confidence and understanding of the world around them. This greater understanding increases the probability that they will not become alienated from society (Boocock & Schild, 1981). Furthermore, simulation games also reduce the gap between the successful and less successful students potentially enhancing the self-confidence of the latter.

It encourages intellectual thought. For example, a game illustrating the complexities of comprehensive health care planning encourages students to acquire skills in personnel planning, working with advisory groups, and interpreting statistics.

Simulation games stimulate student involvement and are fun. Obviously they require more student involvement than merely taking notes. That fact alone may help explain the often high student ratings games receive. Students' increased involvement increases the chances that they will gain insights into the complexities surrounding decisions. Students often prefer them to other classroom activities (Coleman, Livingston, Fennessey, Edwards, & Kidder, 1973).

The games provide a method for teaching through the use of analogies. Analogies are powerful tools that can be used to explain theories. A theory is a hypothesis or generalization about relationships in the world that is descriptive and has high credibility. Through simulation, models can be created that represent the real world. A central characteristic of these models is that they are analogous. Therefore, the value of simulation games is in part their relationship to modeling and analogy. In other words, they help integrate theoretical concepts to simulate real life situations.

Simulation games provide gestalt (that is, they allow students to view issues/problems in their totality).

Learning is facilitated because games provide immediate knowledge of results or feedback. Skinner (1968) criticizes current educational practice by observing that there is too great a time lapse between behavior and knowledge of results. This criticism is invalid for simulation games. Unlike several traditional learning methods, the games provide immediate feedback.

They offer a superior technique for encouraging creative behavior and divergent thought. Torrance (1970) maintains that creative behavior can be encouraged if (1) the instructor's tendency to censor is inhibited, (2) the student is deeply involved, and (3) an unproductive learner comes in close contact with a productive one. Simulation games often meet all these criteria.

Torrence (1970) also suggests creative behavior can be stimulated by (1) the development of a tolerance for complexity and a certain kind of disorder and (2) by incompleteness or a sense that not everything is present. Simulation gaming also often meets these criteria.

Research suggests that simulation games are worthwhile for affective learning (Coleman et al., 1973). It generally is agreed that simulation gaming has its greatest measurable effect in the area of attitudes (Gordon, 1970). Furthermore, when simulation gaming involves role taking, it can change students' attitudes toward the real-life persons whose positions they take (Coleman et al., 1973).

Simulation gaming mirrors real-life experiences. Students vicariously experience some of the doubts and anxieties they would actually face in the clinical setting. This experiential learning seems to be retained longer than information processing (Coleman et al., 1973). However, while simulation gaming does mirror life, the learning environment is protected from the consequences of reality—no "real" harm ever comes to the hypothetical patient.

Limitations of Simulation Gaming

The biggest handicap with simulation games is the amount of class time needed to play them. Objectives that may be implemented using simulation gaming often are not given high priority by instructors. However, students' feedback from simulation gaming methods is very positive. They report increased interest in class, more feeling of involvement in learning, greater ability to transfer theoretical concepts to practice, and less threat in situations similar to those simulated in class (Davidhizar, 1977).

A second criticism is that simulation games may be so complex that the primary concepts and principles are lost to the students. A game's complexity combined with its requirements for active and assertive negotiating behaviors may overwhelm unprepared students. As a result, the primary purpose for playing the game is not achieved.

Simulation games may be so complex (i.e., multidimensional and multievent) that it is impossible for the instructor to monitor all their learning activities. Because of this complexity there is a greater risk that some students may have uncorrected learning experiences (Bernstein, 1977).

REFERENCES

Alexander, L.T., & Abramson, J.H. *Using a discussion to teach: Teaching lab workshop, Small group discussion.* East Lansing, Mich.: Michigan State University Press, 1975.

Allen, D., & Ryan, K. *Microteaching.* Reading, Mass.: Addision-Wesley Publishing Company, Inc., 1969.

Andrews, K.R. (Ed.). *The case method of teaching human relations and administration.* Cambridge, Mass.: Harvard University Press, 1956.

Atkinson, F.D. *List of simulation activities.* Washington, D.C.: Department of Health, Education, and Welfare, National Institutes of Health, National Library of Medicine, Contract No. 1-LM-7-4724, September 1979.

Bandura, A., & Walters, R. *Social learning and personality development.* New York: Holt, Rinehart & Winston, Inc., 1963.

Barnes-McConnell, P.W. Leading discussions. In O. Milton & Associates (Eds.), *On college teaching.* San Francisco: Jossey-Bass, Inc., Publishers, 1978.

Bavelas, A. Role playing and management training. *Sociatry,* 1947, *1,* 183–191.

Berne, E. *Games people play.* New York, Grove Press, 1964.

Bernstein, H.R. Alternative teaching methods. In S.S. Scholl & S.C. Inglis, *Teaching in higher education: Readings for faculty.* Columbus, Ohio: Ohio Board of Regents, 1977.

Boocock, S.S., & Schild, E.O. (Eds.). *Simulation games in learning* (5th printing). Beverly Hills, Calif.: Sage Publications, Inc., 1981.

Bowling, B. *Questioning: The mechanics and dynamics.* Lexington, Ky.: University of Kentucky, Center for Learning Resources, Teaching Improvement Program, n.d.

Bruner, J.S. The act of discovery. *Harvard Educational Review,* 1961, *31,* 21–32.

Clark, C.C. Simulation gaming: A new teaching strategy in nursing education. *Nurse Educator,* 1976, 4–9.

Clore, G.L., & Jeffery, K.M. *Emotional role playing, attitude change and attraction toward a disabled person.* Paper presented at the convention of the Midwestern Psychological Association, Detroit, May 1971.

Coleman, J.S., Livingston, S.A., Fennessey, G.M., Edwards, K.J., & Kidder, S.J. The Hopkins games program: Conclusions from seven years of research. *Educational Research,* 1973, *2*(8), 3–7.

Daniel, E.L. *Any other song: A plea for holistic communications.* Bowie, Md.: Robert J. Brady Company, 1980.

Davidhizar, R.E. Use of simulation games in teaching psychiatric nursing. *Journal of Nursing Education,* 1977, *16*(5), 9–11.

Dewey, J. *Democracy and education.* New York: The Macmillan Company, 1928.

Duke, R. *Gaming: The future's language.* New York: Halsted Press, 1974.

Fisher, C.F. Being there vicariously by case studies. In O. Milton & Associates (Eds.), *On college teaching.* San Francisco: Jossey-Bass, Inc., Publishers, 1978.

Hawley, R.C., & Hawley, I.L. *Human values in the classroom.* New York: Hart Publishing Company, Inc., 1975.

Hill, W.F. *Learning thru discussion.* Beverly Hills, Calif.: Sage Publications, Inc., 1977.

Inbar, M. The differential impact of a game simulating a community disaster and its implications for games with simulated environments. Baltimore, Md.: The Johns Hopkins University Department of Social Relations, 1966. Unpublished doctoral dissertation.

Johnson, W.D. The effects of cognitive closure on learner achievement. (Doctoral dissertation, Stanford University, 1965). *Dissertation Abstracts International,* 1965, University Microfilms No. 65-2861.

King, E. *Classroom evaluation strategies.* St. Louis: The C.V. Mosby Company, 1979.

Kohlberg, L. The cognitive-developmental approach to moral education. *Phi Delta Kappan,* June 1975, *56*(10), 670–677.

Liveright, A. Role playing in leadership training. *Personnel Journal,* 1951, *29,* 412–416.

Maley, D.A. *The industrial arts teacher's handbook.* Boston: Allyn & Bacon, Inc., 1978.

Moore, O.K., & Anderson, A.R. Autotelic folk models. *Sociological Quarterly,* 1960, *1,* 206–216.

Moreno, J.L. *Who shall survive?* New York: Beacon House, 1953.

Piaget, J. *The moral judgment of the child* (2nd ed.). Glencoe, Ill.: The Free Press, 1948.

Rockler, M.J. Applying simulation/gaming. O. Milton & Associates (Eds.), *On college teaching.* San Francisco: Jossey-Bass, Inc., Publishers, 1978.

Rowe, M.B. *Teaching science as continuous inquiry.* New York: McGraw-Hill Book Company, 1978.

Schulman, E.D. *Intervention in human services.* St. Louis: The C.V. Mosby Company, 1974.

Skinner, B.F. *The technology of teaching.* New York: Appleton-Century-Crofts, Inc., 1968.

Stivers, S.N.; Buchan, L.G.; Dettloff, C.R.; & Orlich, D.C. Humanism: Capstone of an educated person. *Clearing House,* 1972, *46,* 556–560.

Taba, H. *Handbook for elementary social studies.* Reading, Mass.: Addison-Wesley Publishing Company, Inc., 1967.

The Herald-Leader, Lexington, Kentucky, 21 June, 1981.

Torrance, E.P. *Encouraging creativity in the classroom.* Dubuque, Iowa: William C. Brown Company Publishers, 1970.

Zaltman, G. *Consumer Game,* Copyright 1966.

Appendix 3-A

Nursing Dilemma Case Studies

Case No.	Summary of Incident	Clinical Area Setting
1.	The nurse is primary therapist for a 16-year-old boy who becomes psychotic after taking some medication smuggled to him by another patient. The team decision was to keep the patient who took the drugs to the Unit on Room Restriction for five days. The nurse strongly recommended this prolonged restriction. This nurse now is being criticized by her peers for being protective of the 16-year-old and punitive to the other patient. She wonders whether she was retaliating, "getting back," meeting her own needs. She wonders whether she should recommend less time for the patient on Room Restriction.	Detoxification Unit General Hospital
2.	A young male patient ran from a supervised group of patients playing volleyball in a park by a river. An orderly ran after him but the patient quickly rolled down the bank and drowned. The nurse had heard this	Psychiatric Unit General Hospital

Source: These cases are adapted from summaries of interviews with professional nurses by Patricia Crisham, R.N., Ph.D., Associate Professor, School of Nursing, University of Minnesota. Copyright © 1978, by permission of the author.

Case No.	Summary of Incident	Clinical Area Setting
	patient express suicidal thoughts that morning but had not communicated this to the recreational therapist who took the patients to the park. The nurse feels guilty. She wonders whether she should tell someone about her earlier encounter with the patient. She wonders whether she should turn in her resignation.	
3.	On the evening shift, a man whose wife delivered a child the day before asks whether he may stay in the same room with his wife tonight. His wife is in a private room. After exploring the situation, the nurse believes it important for this patient and her husband and wants to permit this. However, this would violate hospital policy. The nurse is uncertain what her response should be.	Maternity Unit General Hospital
4.	A 3-year-old child recently was diagnosed as having leukemia. The child's physician wrote an order not to discuss the illness with the family and left town for a week. The mother is asking leading questions about the child's health. The nurse feels an obligation to "carry out the doctor's order" but also wants to respond to the expressed needs of this family.	Pediatrics General Hospital
5.	The evening nurse is about to give a newly ordered drug. She notices that the ordered dosage is abnormally large, confirms this by checking references, and calls the physician. The doctor states that he has ordered what he wants given. The nurse wonders whether she should give the drug.	Intensive Care Unit General Hospital

Case No.	Summary of Incident	Clinical Area Setting
6.	A patient asks the nurse numerous questions about the experimental chemotherapy that has been suggested to the patient by the physician. The nurse is uncertain about the amount of information she should share concerning details as to the action of the drug, positive results noted with other patients, dangerous side effects, etc.	Oncology Unit General Hospital
7.	On a Sunday, the nurse is the only R.N. on duty with 40 acutely ill patients. In making assignments, she struggles to decide whether the patients should be divided equally among the three nurse aides and she herself be available briefly to all patients or whether she should give direct care to the most seriously ill and have the nurse aides provide for the other patients with little or no supervision.	Medical-Surgical Unit General Hospital
8.	A nurse who was hired as a "float nurse" has strong moral objections to abortions. Whenever she is assigned to the unit where abortions are being done, she refuses to go. The nurse wonders whether this is the right thing for her to do.	Maternity Unit General Hospital
9.	A nurse sees another nurse going home with rolls of tape and sterile dressings in her purse. She decides to ignore this but wonders whether the patient is paying for this in the end and whether she should tell someone what she has observed.	Orthopedic Unit General Hospital
10.	At the time of discharge, a patient insists that the nurse take a valuable ring. The patient expresses gratitude	Psychiatric Unit General Hospital

Case No.	Summary of Incident	Clinical Area Setting
	and will not allow the nurse to refuse the ring. The nurse feels she should accept it for the patient's sake but feels guilty about doing so. She is uncertain about what to do.	
11.	An elderly lady has fallen and fractured her hip while attempting to go to the bathroom during the night. The next morning, her husband asks numerous questions about the fall, about the number and type of staff on duty, how long it takes someone to answer a patient's light, etc. The nurse wonders how much information to share with this husband.	Medical Unit General Hospital
12.	A patient asks a nurse whether she believes the patient would be wise in changing therapists. The nurse is convinced that the patient's therapist is inadequate but wonders what she should reply.	Psychiatric Unit General Hospital
13.	At a staff nurse inservice educational program, a transparency is shown with the name and extensive details about a patient who was discharged recently. The nurse feels this violates the patient's right to privacy but is uncertain whether she should initiate action to stop this.	Education Unit General Hospital
14.	A nurse mistakenly gives the wrong medication to a child. She decides it is not serious and does not report or chart it. A few days later, after the child has been discharged, she continues to be concerned about what she did, feels guilty about covering her mistake, and wonders what would happen if she reports this incident now.	Pediatric Unit General Hospital

Case No.	Summary of Incident	Clinical Area Setting
15.	A student tells a faculty member that she is pregnant. School of Nursing regulations state that a student may not begin a semester in clinical courses when she is pregnant. The student says she will be able to hide her pregnancy during the semester and cannot afford to delay completing the program. The faculty member wonders whether she has an obligation to keep this confidential, as the student requested, or to tell the school administration.	School of Nursing
16.	A nurse notices another nurse regularly putting patients' medications in her purse. After experiencing some turmoil about what she should do, the nurse makes an appointment with the head nurse to tell her about this. Nothing changes and the nurse continues to take patients' medications. The nurse who continues to observe this wonders what she should do.	Psychiatric Unit State Hospital
17.	A nurse records inaccurate information on a patient's chart because of a complicated, delicate situation involving a psychiatrist she admires. The situation becomes more complex and now the nurse does not know what she should do.	Psychiatric Unit General Hospital
18.	The evening nurse notices that the inhalation therapist regularly arrives on the unit slightly disoriented and with the odor of alcohol on his breath. The nurse is concerned about the treatment he gives patients but also worries about the consequences if she reports this. The situation is complicated by the fact that the nurse's hus-	Medical Unit General Hospital

Case No.	Summary of Incident	Clinical Area Setting
	band is a good friend of the inhalation therapist.	
19.	A nurse regularly observes serious breaks in technique by another registered nurse. The former feels she should do something about this because of the serious complications that could result from the latter nurse's carelessness. She regularly rationalizes, however, that it is not her responsibility.	Operating Room General Hospital
20.	A nurse is about to add the last IV solution that has been ordered for a man who had surgery two days earlier. The nurse's observations result in her questioning whether this man should have additional fluids. It is 3 a.m. and she knows the surgeon would be very angry if called during the night. She struggles with whether she should be the patient's advocate, call the surgeon, check out what would be best, and possibly not add the fluids. The other alternative is not to call and check, protect the surgeon's sleep, protect herself from his anger, and automatically add the IV solution.	Surgical Unit General Hospital
21.	A 15-year-old boy is brought into the Emergency Room with a spinal cord injury resulting from a diving accident. During this crisis, the nurse is able to establish a helping relationship with his parents. Two days later the parents come to the Emergency Room and tell the nurse that their son will be permanently paralyzed from the neck down and they need to decide at this time whether to take "extraordinary means" to keep him alive. They ask	Emergency Room Children's Hospital

Case No.	Summary of Incident	Clinical Area Setting
	the nurse for "advice." The decision for the nurse is whether to answer their question. She also needs to decide what she believes about prolonging this boy's life with "extraordinary means."	
22.	In home visits to a mother and a newborn, the nurse meets a lethargic 2-year-old son. As she observes this frightened child, seemingly in pain as he moves, she asks the mother about him. The mother's response and the evaluation of the boy result in the nurse's wondering about "child abuse." The nurse wants to communicate her findings to an official authority but fears she may get into serious difficulties for doing so.	Public Health Private Visiting Nurse Association

Appendix 3-B

Selected List of Simulation Activities

Name: *Community Health Worker*
Description: Players in this activity attempt to influence community leaders to accept better methods of health care delivery. This activity helps players become aware of various strategies for delivering community health care services.
Participants: Designed for two to 12 players.
Time: One to two hours.
Cost: Approximately $3.
Source: International Communications Institute
              P.O. Box 8268, Station F
              Edmonton, Alberta
              Canada T 6 H 4 Pi.

Name: *Mental Health*
Description: A card game with role playing in which participants try out techniques used to cope with stress and anxiety in everyday conflicts and problems. The goal of the game is to win by protecting basic needs and acquiring coping cards to reduce or eliminate stress and anxiety.
Participants: Designed for two to six players.
Time: One to three hours.
Cost: Approximately $9.
Source: Union Printing Co., Inc.
              17 West Washington Street
              Athens, Ohio 45701

Source: Selected from a compilation by F.D. Atkinson for the Department of Health, Education, and Welfare, National Institutes of Health, National Library of Medicine, Contract No. 1-LM-7-4724, September, 1979.

Name: *The Ungame*
Description: A noncompetitive activity in which the players learn how to communicate more effectively as they share thoughts, ideas, and feelings. A game board, die, and cards determine the progress of the activity.
Participants: Designed for two to six players.
Time: Determined by players, with a suggested duration of one hour.
Cost: Approximately $10.
Comments: An interesting noncompetitive activity with format that could be adapted to deal with many health science education issues.
Source: The Ungame Company
               1440 South State College Boulevard
               Anaheim, Calif. 92806

Name: *Where Do You Draw the Line?*
Description: A simulation activity designed to involve the participants in a discussion of ethical issues and values. Players make judgments as to the acceptability of the behavior of individuals, corporations, and organizations as described in a series of vignettes. Included are a director's guide, decision forms, response markers, situation forms, summary of situations, and a transparency to summarize the group's decisions.
Participants: Designed for any age group concerned with discussing ethics or values. Five to 35 participants may participate in teams or individually.
Time: Usually one hour.
Cost: Approximately $20.
Comments: Excellent model of nonconsumable forms, interactive procedures, and a very complete director's guide.
Source: Simile II
               Box 910
               Del Mar, Calif. 92014

Name: *Into Aging*
Description: A simulation game intended to dramatize certain attitudes and beliefs underlying society's way of dealing with the elderly. Players assume the identity of an old person with certain goals and obtain rewards and penalties, depending on their actions. The ultimate goal is that players' per-

spective and orientation toward the elderly will become more positive.

Participants:	Designed for five to 15 players. Intended for anyone who deals with the aging, such as health professionals, educators, and families with elderly members.
Time:	Approximately two hours.
Cost:	Approximately $12.
Comments:	This simulation game contains particularly good examples of an effective leader's guide and very clear players' directions. Procedures can be readily adapted to their content areas.
Source:	Charles B. Slack, Inc. Thorofare, N.J. 08086

Name:	*Psychiatric Nurse-Patient Relationship Game*
Description:	A highly programmed role-playing activity that simulates the orientation, working, and termination phases of the nurse-patient relationship.
Participants:	Designed primarily for psychiatric nursing students. Two players are required, one taking the role of learner and the other that of teacher.
Time:	Approximately three hours, depending upon the skill of the players.
Cost:	Approximately $18.
Comments:	An interesting example of an activity designed to be conducted with little intervention by the instructor. Many of the procedures and evaluation forms could be adapted for use in other content areas.
Source:	Carolyn Chambers Clark P.O. Box 132 Sloatsburg, N.Y. 10974

Name:	*Circulation*
Description:	A board game that deals with some of the basic concepts related to the human circulatory system. Components include a game board, white blood cells, plasma trays, oxygen discs, food squares, waste squares, emergency cards, circulatory cards, and a game spinner.
Participants:	Designed for two to four players.
Time:	Usually 30 to 60 minutes.
Cost:	Approximately $15.

Comments: A very worthwhile board game to play and critique to determine what elements could be adapted and/or improved to teach other basic health science concepts.

Source: Teaching Concepts, Inc.
230 Park Avenue
New York, N.Y. 10017

Name: *Futuribles*

Description: A game consisting of 288 cards, each citing a future probability in areas such as communication, energy, food, human experience, learning, religion, etc. Participants become familiar with a variety of forecasts and become aware of their personal feelings and responsibility for the future.

Participants: Designed for any number of players in groups of six to eight members.

Time: Varies widely, depending upon the players and the particular version being played—can last from 15 minutes to four hours or more.

Cost: Approximately $10.

Comments: An excellent model of a card game that is highly interactive and noncompetitive and that can be played successfully with no special content expertise. It also provides an example of how one basic set of cards can be used in a variety of levels from very simple to quite complex.

Source: Service Department, Board of Discipleship
The United Methodist Church
Local Church Education
P.O. Box 840
Nashville, Tenn. 37202

Name: *Super-Sandwich*

Description: A board game in which players go to breakfast, lunch, and dinner as they purchase a wide variety of foods to meet their recommended dietary allowances of calories, protein, vitamins, and minerals. Players learn the basic facts of nutrition.

Participants: Designed for two to four players.

Time: Usually 30 to 60 minutes.

Cost: Approximately $15.

Source: Teaching Concepts, Inc.
230 Park Avenue
New York, N.Y. 10017

Name: *The Drug Debate*

Description: A highly interactive instrument that involves role-playing competition between teams and cooperation within teams. The debate is structured so that opposing points of view must be presented and given serious consideration. Eight drugs must be discussed, with no attempt to promote a particular point of view.

Participants: Designed for eight or more players in 2 to 16 teams.

Time: Varies from two to seven hours.

Cost: Approximately $30.

Source: Academic Games Associates, Inc.
430 East 33rd Street
Baltimore, Md. 21218

Name: *The O K Game*

Description: This board game is designed to help players become aware of the way they communicate with others. The concepts, terminology, and roles are clearly drawn from the transactional analysis field.

Participants: Designed for two to six players.

Time: Thirty to 60 minutes.

Cost: Approximately $10.

Source: Simco Enterprises
3012 Samoa Place
Costa Mesa, Calif. 92626

Name: *Reunion*

Description: A noncompetitive activity that involves sharing memories, feelings, imaginings, and intuition. A spinner, die, cards, and game board determine who shares what types of information.

Participants: Designed for two to six players.

Time: Determined by players, usually is one hour or longer.

Cost: Approximately $10.

Comments: An excellent model of a noncompetitive game in which the board is simply a way of determining who shares what type of information. Particularly useful for those interested in team building, group dynamics, and interpersonal relations.

Source: The Ungame Company
1440 South State College Boulevard
Anaheim, Calif. 92806

Related Publications

A Handbook of Structured Experiences for Human Relations Training,
Vols. 1, 2, 3, 4, 5, 6, 7. J.W. Pfieffer & J.E. Jones (Eds.). La Jolla, Calif.:
University Associates, Inc., 1979.

Seven volumes consist of easy-to-use structured group activities. These
activities, described in thorough detail, are designed for use in planning,
trust building, cooperation, consensus, getting acquainted, group problem
solving, leadership, competition, and intergroup communication. Many of
these procedures can be incorporated into the design of activities directly
related to health science education.

The Annual Handbook for Group Facilitators. 1972, 1973, 1974, 1975,
1976, 1977, 1978, 1979, 1980, J.W. Pfeiffer & J.E. Jones (Eds.). La Jolla,
Calif.: University Associates, Inc.

The annuals contain collections of structural experiences. Many of the
procedures can be adapted to health science education.

The Guide to Simulations/Games for Education and Training, Vols. 1, 2
(3rd ed.), Robert Horn (Ed.). Cranford, N.J.: Didactic Systems, Inc.,
1977. Cost: Approximately $25.

The guide contains approximately 700 pages of simulation game descriptions in all content areas.

Appendix 3-C

Simulation Game Example*

"The Kidney Machine Problem"

Objectives

1. To develop an increased awareness of one's own value system.
2. To develop awareness that different people have—and act upon— different values.

Group Size and Physical Setting

A large class should be divided into small groups of seven to nine students. These groups should be organized into small circles so that everyone can see each other.

Time Required

Two to two and a half hours.

Process

1. The facilitator introduces "the Kidney Machine Problem" by discussing the objectives of the activity and reading the introduction to the game and the specific directions.

Note: Kidney dialysis has become increasingly available. However, it is still time consuming and expensive. The emotional problems experienced by patients dependent on the machine are still the same. The exercise can also be adapted for use with problems associated with other new medical technology.

Source: Adapted from "Kidney Machine: Group Decision Making" by Gerald M. Phillips in J.W. Pfeiffer & J.E. Jones (Eds.), *The 1974 Annual Handbook for Group Facilitators*, pp. 78–87. Used with permission of Gerald M. Phillips, professor of speech communications, Pennsylvania State University.

2. The facilitator notes that in solving the problem, no group votes can be taken. The objective is to reach consensus—defined as substantial agreement, not unanimity.
3. The facilitator leads a debriefing discussion after the groups have selected the individuals to be assigned to vacancies on the machine.

The following questions can be posed by the facilitator during the debriefing:

1. How different were the values within your group?
2. How did your personal value system affect your decision?
3. Do you feel that the conflicting values affected the decision?
4. Do you feel that each member listened fairly to your ideas?
5. Do you listen with an open mind to the ideas of others?
6. Do you believe that you were attacked personally at any point during the discussion?
7. Did you feel like withdrawing from the group at any time?
8. How do you feel toward the other members, now that the activity has ended?
9. How satisfied are you with the decisions that were reached by the group?

The Kidney Machine Problem

At the Swedish Hospital in Seattle, the world-famous kidney machine is a social curiosity. It saves lives in a most peculiar way. Some people suffer from a relatively rare kidney disease, which without the kidney machine is fatal. Today, a very expensive piece of equipment can keep people who have this machine alive. Of course, there are not enough opportunities to get at the machine to service everyone who needs it. For the purposes of this exercise only seven people can be served. There are many more who seek the service.

At present, a number of foundations are raising money for service to people suffering from the disease. One foundation, for example, has made it possible for any person who has access to the kidney machine to be treated without charge. Consequently, while money is a major consideration, it will not be a primary deterrent for using the machine. Another foundation is busily trying to raise funds to purchase another machine. It is getting close to its objective but is not there yet.

Medical science can make a very accurate prognosis of who can profit from use of the machine. The medical decision, in fact, is quite easy to make, so, again, the doctors have a long list of people who could remain alive if they had access to the machine. The decision about who is serviced has to be made on criteria other than medical.

Swedish Hospital has solved this problem by appointing a volunteer citizens panel, ordinary people like you and me, to decide who should be served and who should not. They make their decisions on simple information. They are given a factual profile of medically eligible candidates and a psychologist's report that tells them something about the personality of potential subjects. The panel then meets, discusses the people, and makes a decision based on a consensus (not vote) about who should be assigned as a patient to be served by the machine.

The panel members decide in their own way. They are not observed and they are not questioned. They meet, they talk, they decide, and they report their decision. They never meet the candidates; they do not see their pictures. In fact, members of the panel are strangers to each other when they first come together and they do not see each other except when they serve on the panel. They have the following basic criteria to consider:

1. People between the ages of 20 and 40 seem to have the best prognosis for a satisfactory life if served by the machine.
2. There is considerable potential for emotional disturbance in patients on the machine. They become dependent on the service and can become sullen and resentful. Some have been known to become very belligerent to the doctors and nurses who supply the service.
3. For those selected, money is no object.

Instructions to Students:

Your problem is to examine the information about the ten individuals included here and to determine which two of them should be assigned to vacancies on the machine. You should read the information carefully and make whatever decisions you care to.

Next, your group should meet and devise the method that you will use to make your decision.

Finally, you should select your two people and prepare a report that explains your choice and includes the criteria that guided the decision. Present this report to your instructor.

1. **Norman D.** (White, male, American)

Age 31. Occupation: Insurance underwriter. Wife (30, employed as a secretary in the office of the company for which her husband worked). Son (6, student in elementary school). Also caring for Mrs. D. (Norman's mother) who was ill. Held B.B.A. degree from midwestern university.

Family income: $39,600 per year ($24,000 from husband, $12,000 from wife, and the rest Social Security payments to Mrs. D.).

Personality Profile

Mr. D. expressed distress about his lot in life. He told the panel that he had hoped for a lot more when he graduated from college, and described in vivid detail what it was like to be a 9-to-5 man in the office of a large insurance company. He talked about his dreams of going to a warm place to write poetry and showed the panel some of the poetry he had written in his spare time. The panel agreed that the poetry was certainly expressive of his inner disturbance but no member was qualified to determine whether or not Mr. D. showed promise as a writer.

Mr. D. told the panel that he intended to write a daily journal of his feelings from now until the end in the hope that it could be published and the proceeds given as a legacy to his wife. He expressed considerable concern about the financial future of his family and told the panel several times that "there is no one else to help." He became very involved in a discussion of the plight of the middle-class American, with no one concerned about his welfare, and condemned the government for its activities on behalf of "people who really don't want to work and who just take the jobs from people who want to get ahead."

Mr. D. was heavily involved in the activities of a political-religious Protestant church group and also was a campaign worker for the democratic presidential candidate. Mr. D. asserted that if he were permitted to live he would attempt to implement a cherished dream of entering politics and trying to make some important changes in the world.

2. **Clark B.** (White, male, Mexican National)

Age 24. Occupation: Stevedore. Wife (17, not employed). Daughter (6 months). No education shown on record. Not literate. Family income: $8,000 per year.

Personality Profile

Mr. B. came to the area with his wife about six months ago, just before their baby was born. They had been working as migrant farm laborers. When the baby was born he sought and found permanent employment in the area. He hoped that he would be able to work "for a long time, until the child is grown," but he also expressed a dim view of his future since he was "not learned and not able to learn." The panel suggested commitment to a program of vocational training in the local community college and that he make an attempt to acquire literacy through the general educational development program but he did not appear to be interested in either.

Mr. B. spent a good deal of time before the committee inquiring about the availability of charitable services for his wife and child in the event of his death and made it quite clear to the panel that he did not expect that "someone like me would be picked to stay alive."

3. **Carter P.** (White, male, American)

Age 30. Occupation: Self-employed (owner of public relations firm, free-lance author). Wife (20, employed as night club entertainer). No children. Held B.S. degree in engineering from eastern university. Family income: Approximately $1 million (wife's share, about $55,000).

Personality Profile

Mr. P. was hardnosed and almost a stereotype of the entrepreneur. He had little financial backing when he graduated from college. He started as a human relations consultant to industry and rapidly built his public relations consulting firm into one of the largest on the West Coast. He devoted a great deal of time to consultation on issues of community concern and at the time of the interview was in charge of the governor's campaign against air and water pollution. He pointed with pride to his filmed commercials that were shown on most television stations in the area.

He was proud of his wife. They had been married for less than a year. She was a singer in a local night club. He had met her in Las Vegas and declared with pride that he married her within a week. They were planning to build a home in a northern mountain area, which they characterized as their retreat. She also appeared to support his community action projects.

Colleagues of Mr. P. regarded him as a man of high ethical principles and were unanimous in their praise of his skill at his profession. He declared that if permitted to live, he knew he would "have the power to do something that matters in this society." He stipulated as a goal, "the total elimination of air and water pollution in this community to set a model for other communities all over the country to follow." He notified the panel that win, lose, or draw, he would contribute an amount equivalent to his care cost to one of the fund-raising foundations and also indicated that he had devoted a segment of his firm to consulting in fund raising with the foundations at no cost to them.

4. **John W.** (White, male, American)

Age 39. Occupation: physician, instructor in medical school. Wife (age 35, not employed). Son (15, student in high school), son (13, in junior high school, daughter (9, in elementary school), son (6, student in school for the mentally retarded). Held B.A. and M.D. degrees. Family income: $154,000 per year, contributed entirely by husband.

Personality Profile

John W. had been working with a medical team at the university hospital on a cancer research project. He seemed very involved in the project and asserted that he was "on the verge of a major breakthrough in cancer detection." His colleagues regarded him as a very competent, brilliant colleague but somewhat impatient, volatile, and a little difficult when working with groups.

Relations with his wife had not been good recently. Since the birth of their last son, there had been considerable talk of divorce but both parties agreed that it would be wise to keep the family together in the interest of the children. There was no outward hostility in the home, but the parents had little contact with each other. John W. was active in youth activities, particularly in Boy Scouts and Little League. He was a member of a suburban Rotary Club. Subject appeared to have little contact with his daughter. Wife was active in various charitable groups and civic organizations and was an officer in the local chapter of the League of Women Voters. Some of John W.'s colleagues alleged that he had been active in right-to-life issues and that he opposed abortion for any reason.

John W. had received several honors for his medical research. Two years ago he had been named by the American Medical Association as one of the ten best research physicians in the country. His advancement in the university had been rapid. He had published ten articles in medical journals, most of which had received a high evaluation.

He seemed very anxious to be served by the machine. He impressed the panel as being very dedicated to his work, almost to the exclusion of other considerations, and the panel felt that he would be very productive if permitted to continue.

5. **Warren G.** (White, male, American)

Age 36. Occupation: Rabbi. Wife (34, not employed). Daughter (6, student in elementary school), son (3). Held B.A. degree and D.D. from theological seminary. Family income: $55,000 ($40,000 from husband, $15,000 endowment income from wife's legacy).

Personality Profile

Rabbi G. had been heading his present congregation for six years, joining it directly from military service as a chaplain. It was a new congregation when he took it over and he built it steadily from a 50-family group to its present 470 families. He was to preside over the opening of the new synagogue next month.

His congregants regarded him as an inspiring leader and pointed with pride to his skill as a community builder and fund raiser. The congregation had offered him a life contract. His wife was active in religious activities, worked with the congregation's women's organization, and served as a teacher in the afternoon Hebrew school. She was an Israeli by birth and was raising her two children bilingually. She and the children had spent the last two summers in Israel while her husband enrolled for courses in the Division of American Studies at the local university.

Rabbi G. appeared to be a self-contained, almost austere man. He seemed to take his illness as a matter of fact and expressed to the panel an attitude of "what will be, will be." He asked questions about other possible candidates, expressing his willingness to lend his support to those "worth saving," but the committee, of course, kept such information confidential. He discussed with the committee, at length, the possible merits of having people now assigned to the kidney machine serve on the selection committee. "These people," he said, "would have greater insight into the kind of person that would profit most from being kept alive—the person who gives the most in return for the gift of life." The panel assured him that there were good reasons why current patients did not serve on the committee.

6. Aretha N. (Black, female, American)

Age 22. Occupation: supervisor of neighborhood community center. Divorced (former husband now in prison). No children. B.A. graduate in social work. Income: $14,000 per year.

Personality Profile

Ms. N. was a committed black activist. She functioned under the name of Selima X and claimed membership in the Muslims' auxiliary organization. Her current program sought to build psychological strength into black elementary school children. She also directed a program in literacy training for teenagers and young adults in her community center.

She talked at length with the panel about her goals for her people and seemed quite selfless in her outlook. She conveyed the strength and passion of a real leader and, although she was frankly hostile to whites, she still seemed to be in a frame of mind that would permit her to deal honestly with the white community. She explained to the panel that there were a few white people working with her community center that she trusted completely and knew that they would be the bridge between the races.

She sometimes talked of separatism but most of the time seemed to be realistic in her assessment of the future course of the black community.

She seemed angry, almost paranoid, about her physical condition, as though it were some kind of plot by the community. She refused to meet with the panel twice on the ground that it included no black psychologists. She finally appeared when the interview team was augmented with two black colleagues. Before speaking to the rest of the members, she cross-examined them about their attitudes on racial questions and did not really submit to interview until she was satisfied with them.

7. **Melvin K.** (White, male, American)

Age 19. Student: Junior (philosophy) at local university. Father (age 44, owner of a men's clothing store), mother (deceased for four years), sister (14, student in junior high school), sister (10, in elementary school).

Personality Profile

Melvin appeared to be a sincere young activist. He had been involved in protest demonstrations, including spending one night in jail. He had and expressed deep convictions about the plight of man, particularly about the military buildup and the threat of nuclear war. He expressed the hope that he might be able to seek an advanced degree in philosophy and work with young people. He also displayed some ambiguity when he informed the panel that his father wanted him to be a lawyer and his mother had encouraged him toward a career in medicine. He was engaged to a student (age 18) and said that her father (an industrialist) was encouraging him to transfer into the school of business so Melvin could work at his plant after graduation.

Melvin had little contact with his family even though he attended college in his home town. His sisters informed the panel that he spent little time talking to them and seemed either to treat them brusquely or not even to recognize they were around. He was very intense as he talked about his political commitment, and showed little sense of humor. In commenting about his illness, he said, "To die now might be better than to live, considering the direction the world is moving," but in almost the same breath he declared, "I'd hate to be denied my chance to do something about the world. I don't mean to be arrogant but maybe I'm the one who will have the idea that works. It would be so frustrating to die before finding out."

The panel believed that Melvin was fairly typical of the best university students. His grades were good and his professors felt that he would have no trouble getting into graduate school. They were prepared to help him because of his intellectual qualities although they were unanimous in characterizing him as humorless and excessively serious.

8. **Preston C.** (Black, male, American)

Age 29. Occupation: garage mechanic. Wife (age 25, employed as legal secretary), son (6, elementary school student), son (3). Withdrew from school in eighth grade and took training in night vocational-technical program (manpower training program). Family income: $21,000 ($13,000 from wife, $8,000 from husband).

Personality Profile

Mr. C. was deeply devoted to his family. He was attending courses in night school, hoping, he said, "to get enough skill to open my own garage." Although he listed his occupation as "garage mechanic" he only greased cars. His employer was somewhat concerned about his capability to do anything more complicated.

His children were in the care of his wife's mother, who lived with them. His wife also was working on an advancement program and was taking courses at business college. Mr. C. was involved in some community activities, particularly youth work. He participated in a recreation program at the local community center. He said, "I want no part of political activities, I just want to make a good living." He also was active in church work and his minister had no reservations about calling him "a good family man."

The panel was convinced that he was a good and honest man and an example to the people of his neighborhood. The panel also was convinced that he would not rise above his current position and that there was some potential of trouble between him and his wife as she continued to acquire professional skills.

He appeared not to realize the severity of his illness. The panel was sure that he did not recognize this decision as crucial to his survival.

9. **Katherine F.** (White, female, American)

Age 36. Occupation: Executive secretary to president of large corporation. Not married. Graduate of business college. Took special training in legal stenography and computer operation. Income $17,000 per year.

Personality Profile

Miss F. was the pride of her office. Everyone who worked with her talked of her indispensability and her boss was the first to admit it. "Good women like her are hard to come by!" he declared. Miss F. had a reputation in her office of being a warm, earnest woman yet she was efficient and kept things moving. The panel regarded her as being a genuine professional at her work.

During her interview, Miss F. indicated that she never had been very interested in marriage and confessed to a brief and unsatisfying Lesbian relationship while in her early twenties. She had dated a bit in high school but had had no such social contact with men since her graduation. She was interested in musical activities and sang lead with the local choral society. She was working on the Christmas production of Handel's "Messiah," which she was directing and singing lead. She also had been active in charitable work and was serving as a teacher on weekends in a Head Start program.

She seemed to be adjusted to her problem. She indicated to the panel that she had no qualms about dying provided that her body could make some contribution to medical research. She planned to donate her body to the medical school. At one point she volunteered to withdraw from consideration for a place on the machine to "simplify the judgment for the people who are confronted with that horrible task."

10. **Laura T.** (White, female, American)

Age 34. Occupation: housewife. Husband (age 37, employed as bartender), son (16, student in high school), daughter (15, in high school), daughter (13, in junior high school), daughter (12, in junior high school), son (10, in elementary school), son (3), again pregnant. Had high school diploma. Family income: $22,000 per year, provided entirely by husband.

Personality Profile

Mrs. T. stated that her goal was to be an "ideal Catholic mother." She seemed inordinately devoted to her children but was not terribly perceptive of her husband's problems in providing for a family of that size. She appeared to have no outside interests or activities. She had enrolled last year in a flower-arranging course but dropped out halfway through because "it took too much time away from the children."

She was terribly distressed by her illness. She already had arranged for her mother-in-law to move in and take care of the children and she had been spending a good deal of time in bed even though the testimony of the physicians seemed to indicate that she need not do this.

She expressed to the panel serious fears about how her family would get on without her and requested urgently that they be taken into account more than her. The panel's attempts to get information from the children about relations with their mother were thwarted by Mrs. T.'s unwillingness to submit to an in-the-home interview. It was the feeling of the panel that there would be considerable hardship in the home if Mrs. T. were to die.

Chapter 4

Construction of Assessment Instruments

The fault is not in using crude measures but in doing nothing until perfection comes along.

R.F. Mager

Nursing instructors are confronted with the often overwhelming and frustrating task of assessing affective behaviors. How do they determine the behaviors to measure? Will categorization of measurement instruments make decisions easier? How do they decrease the influence of drawing inferences?

This chapter presents four orientations to affective assessment: (1) the psychometric, (2) the behavioral, (3) the counseling (Gordon, 1978), and (4) traditional evaluation methods. Each has unique strengths and weaknesses but together they offer worthwhile help with the needed yet difficult task of affective assessment.

The psychometric approach assumes that attitudes and values are psychological constructs that can be measured by responses to test stimuli. The results of these tests provide specific measurement indexes that can be quantified and compared. It involves the use and development of the Likert Scale, the Semantic Differential Scale, and the Thurstone Scale. The major strength of these instruments is that they can help students and faculty gain information that may be unavailable otherwise. However, their results can be faked easily. Students may report only what they believe to be socially acceptable behaviors.

Behavioral orientation is rooted in Skinner's (1969) concept of behaviorism in which much of human behavior is measurable in concrete, objectively observable action. Skinner's theory assumes that behavior also is changeable. Changes in behavior can occur through a skillful program of reinforcement. Behavioral/observational instruments (i.e., rating scales, checklists, and anecdotal records) can be useful. One of their major strengths

141

is that they clarify faculty expectations and communicate them to students (Gordon, 1978). Their use improves consistency of assessment and decreases the use of inference. Documentation of specific behaviors can be made that enables students and faculty to monitor behavior changes. However, the instruments may be time consuming and difficult to develop.

Proponents of the counseling approach to the assessment of affective objectives view the faculty's role in the assessment of affect as helping the students develop insights into their own behavior and personality. It assumes that they are more likely to change behavior and attitudes if they more fully understand themselves. Exploring concepts such as warmth, caring, and stress can help students adapt professional behaviors. The interview is another way for faculty and students to mutually explore perceptions and values that influence observable behaviors. Such discussions can provide the support for constructive behavioral change.

The basic strength of the counseling orientation is that it provides a safe, unconditionally accepting environment in which students are free to risk revealing inadequacies or failures in their attempts to develop professionally acceptable behaviors. However, some faculty members may not be prepared to assume the counselor role.

As for adapting traditional evaluation methods to the assessment of affective objectives, a primary strength of the use of this older approach is that it builds upon knowledge of tests and measurement that are familiar to most educators.

The variety of evaluation methods presented in this chapter reflects the complex nature of both nursing practice and the assessment of it. Instructors can use the methods discussed to diversify their evaluation strategies.

PSYCHOMETRIC ORIENTATION TO ATTITUDES

The word "attitude" may be used to define the sum of individuals' feelings, prejudices, ideas, fears, and beliefs concerning any selected topic. Thus, a woman's attitude about death may encompass all she thinks and feels about living and dying; obviously, it will be quite subjective and personal.

The concept of "opinion" describes an expression of an attitude. For example if a woman states that a serious mistake was made when abortion was legalized, her comment is an expressed opinion. Furthermore the inference to be drawn from her expressed opinion is that she is antiabortion. Consequently, an opinion often reflects an attitude.

The concept of attitude is a complex psychological construct. For example, instead of merely assessing a student's performance on a specific test, the instructor may want to determine that individual's attitude toward psychiatric patients. This hypothetical quality is called a "construct." Educators assume the existence of constructs so they can account for behavior in many specific situations; thus, it may be appropriate to attempt to measure them.

This section provides guidelines for constructing three types of attitude scales:

1. The Likert Scale
2. The Semantic Differential Scale
3. The Thurstone Scale.

In addition, the limitations of attitude measures are analyzed.

THE LIKERT SCALE

The Likert-type scale is the most popular and commonly used attitude assessment instrument. It is relatively easy to construct and requires fewer assumptions than other scaling models. It also has been referred to as "summative scaling" (because the final score is determined by merely adding weighted integers) and "an agreement scale" (since respondents are asked to indicate their agreement with a statement on a five-point scale). The most significant feature of Likert's (1932) scaling is that it assumes that an attitude can be assessed by summing the number of pro or anti opinion statements a person is willing to endorse.

The most common method of constructing a Likert scale is to gather a set of extreme attitude statements that are written to clearly indicate favorable or unfavorable positions. The most relevant opinion statements are sorted into favorable and unfavorable (trying to include an equal number of each) and administered to a group of respondents who are instructed to indicate their agreement/disagreement on a five-point scale.

The major concern is to select items that represent extremes of the attitude to be assessed. Likert scaling assumes that an attitude can be assessed by counting the number of statements for or against opinions an individual is willing to endorse.

Constructing a Likert-Type Scale

In developing a Likert-type scale, the following guidelines can be helpful. The instructor should:

1. determine the attitude variable to be measured
2. accumulate a large number of very favorable or very unfavorable

statements relative to the attitude, value, or feeling to be measured
3. pretest the items on individuals similar to the respondents whose attitudes will be measured
4. identify high scorers (top (25 percent) and low scorers (bottom 25 percent))
5. analyze each attitude statement by determining how well it discriminates between high and low scores; this is called item analysis and is discussed later
6. select and retain attitude statements that can discriminate between high and low scorers; try to select for the final scale 20 to 25 items, half of which should be favorable and half unfavorable
7. construct the Likert-type attitude scale using the items with the best discrimination power
8. administer the instrument (Table 4-1).

Table 4-1 A Sample Likert-Type Scale

Attitudes toward Affiliation Agreements

Directions:
The best answer to each of the following statements is your personal opinion. There are five possible responses for each statement.
SA (Strongly Agree)
 A (Agree)
 U (Undecided)
 D (Disagree)
SD (Strongly Disagree)
Please circle only one of the five responses.

1. The affiliation agreement strengthens the relationship between two parties.	SA	A	U	D	SD
2. The affiliation agreement serves as a guide for clinical education.	SA	A	U	D	SD
3. The affiliation agreement is valuable only if you don't trust the other party.	SA	A	U	D	SD
4. The affiliation agreement is a nuisance.	SA	A	U	D	SD
5. The affiliation agreement is a very important document.	SA	A	U	D	SD
6. I feel very comfortable about writing, reviewing, and/or signing an affiliation agreement.	SA	A	U	D	SD
7. If I had my way, we would have *no* written affiliation agreements.	SA	A	U	D	SD
8. The time spent in negotiating with a clinical center is out of proportion to the benefits.	SA	A	U	D	SD

When the respondents have completed the items, their responses are scored using a system of integer weights developed by Likert (1932). Favorable statements are scored as follows: SA = 5, A = 4, U = 3, D = 2, SD = 1.

The reverse order is used for unfavorable statements: SA = 1, A = 2, U = 3, D = 4, SD = 5.

For the example in Table 4-1, the scoring is shown in Table 4-2. Items 1, 2, 5, and 6 all are favorable and are given weights 5, 4, 3, 2, 1, respectively. In contrast, items 3, 4, 7, and 8 all are unfavorable and are scored in reverse, 1, 2, 3, 4, 5. A respondent who is extremely favorable toward affiliation agreements would respond "Strongly Agree" to items 1, 2, 5, and 6 (20 points) and "Strongly Disagree" with items 3, 4, 7, and 8 (20 points). As a result, a score of 40 points would be interpreted to indicate a very favorable attitude toward affiliation agreements.

Responses to items 1 through 10 in Table 4-3 together constitute a measure of occupational stress. A respondent who is experiencing a high degree of job-related stress probably would respond "always" to statements 1, 2, 5, 7, and 9 and "never" to statements 3, 4, 6, 8, and 10. As a result, a score of 50 would be interpreted to indicate high occupational stress, a score of 10 extremely low job-related stress.

Item analysis procedures can be used to measure how well an attitude statement can discriminate between high and low scorers. The primary purpose of completing an item analysis is to select entries with the highest discrimination index.

If computer services are available, they can provide a more accurate analysis than can be computed by hand and in much less time. However, if they are not available, the following procedure can be used to provide item analysis data for a small pilot group (i.e., 20 to 40 respondents). The instructor should:

Table 4-2 Scoring a Likert-Type Scale

			SA	A	U	D	SD
1.	Item 1	Strongly favorable	5	4	3	2	1
2.	Item 2	Strongly favorable	5	4	3	2	1
3.	Item 3	Strongly unfavorable	1	2	3	4	5
4.	Item 4	Strongly unfavorable	1	2	3	4	5
5.	Item 5	Strongly favorable	5	4	3	2	1
6.	Item 6	Strongly favorable	5	4	3	2	1
7.	Item 7	Strongly unfavorable	1	2	3	4	5
8.	Item 8	Strongly unfavorable	1	2	3	4	5

Table 4-3 Another Type of Likert Scale

Attitudes toward Job Stress

Directions:
The best answer to each of the following statements is your personal opinion. There are five possible responses for each statement.
1 = never
2 = rarely
3 = sometimes
4 = frequently
5 = always
Please circle only one of the five responses.
Describe the extent to which you as supervisor experience the following:

1. Feeling that the amount of work I have to do may interfere with how well the work gets done.	1	2	3	4	5
2. Feeling that I have too heavy a workload, one that can't possibly be finished in an ordinary workday.	1	2	3	4	5
3. Feeling that I can get information needed to carry out my job.	5	4	3	2	1
4. Thinking that I'll be able to satisfy the conflicting demands of various people over me.	5	4	3	2	1
5. Feeling that I'm not fully qualified to handle my job.	1	2	3	4	5
6. Knowing just what the people I work with expect of me.	5	4	3	2	1
7. Having to make decisions that affect the lives of individuals I know.	1	2	3	4	5
8. Feeling that I have enough authority to carry out the responsibilities assigned to me.	5	4	3	2	1
9. Not knowing what administration thinks of me and how my performance is evaluated.	1	2	3	4	5
10. Feeling that my job rarely interferes with my personal life.	5	4	3	2	1

1. arrange all papers from highest to lowest, based upon total score.
2. divide the papers into the half with the highest scores and the half with the lowest, keeping all papers in descending order (if there is an odd number of respondents, discard the middle paper).
3. use a sample work sheet such as that in Table 4-4 and put the total score of each paper in the left-hand column, beginning at the top with the paper that has the highest score; when the highest 50 percent has been tested, jump to the lower half of the table and list the lowest 50 percent.

4. record an *X* under each option selected on the highest paper; the Xs for each paper will run horizontally across the graph. For example, the highest score was 40, and the respondent with that total chose ''Strongly Agree'' for Item 1.
5. record all the responses, then simply count vertically the number of Xs tabulated under each response alternative for the high 50 percent and for the low 50 percent; space to record these data is provided above each item number.

If the response patterns of high and low scores are extremely different, the item is a good discriminating one. For example, Item 1 in Table 4-4 easily discriminates between the high and low scorers. Three of the high scorers responded ''Agree'' and two ''Strongly Agree.'' Four of the low scorers answered ''Strongly Disagree'' and one ''Disagree.'' In contrast, for Item 2, patterns of high and low respondents are identical; consequently, the item cannot discriminate between high and low scores and should be discarded.

Validity and Reliability of Likert Scaling

The most difficult problem with the validity of this technique is the interpretation of the neutral point (Lemon, 1973). Respondents may obtain intermediate scores on scales of this kind by checking the midpoints of

Table 4-4 Work Sheet for Manually Tabulating Item Analysis

		Item #1					Item #2				
High 50%		2	3	0	0	0	2	3	0	0	0
Low 50%		0	0	0	1	4	2	3	0	0	0
	Score:	SA	A	U	D	SD	SA	A	U	D	SD
Upper 50%											
1. Kelly	40	X					X				
2. Kristan	39	X						X			
3. Amy	35		X					X			
4. Janet	35		X				X				
5. Marie	30		X					X			
Lower 50%											
1. Rebecca	25				X		X				
2. Diane	24				X			X			
3. Stephanie	20				X			X			
4. Joel	15			X			X				
5. David	5				X			X			

the agreement scales all the way down or by checking opposite extremes (Table 4-5). While that should not occur with a well-developed scale, the possibility exists.

The reliability of the scale can be determined by the test/retest method or by preparing two parallel forms from the same material and presenting both to the same individual.

Another sample Likert-type scale is shown in Appendix 4-A.

THE SEMANTIC DIFFERENTIAL SCALE

Charles E. Osgood, a psychologist from the University of Illinois, in 1952 proposed to have identified three components of meaning: evaluation, activity, and potency. Data from his conclusions were obtained by asking individuals to rate a series of concepts using a large number of adjective pairs. These sets of adjective pairs are called semantic differential scales.

The semantic differential is a measurement technique used to determine direction of attitude, which is decided by students' selection of polar terms.

The semantic differential usually consists of a number of adjective pairs separated by a seven-point scale. Osgood, Suci, & Tannenbaum (1957) report that seven scale points are about optimum and that fewer divisions irritate respondents while more divisions produce unsatisfactory distributions. Most researchers use scales with an uneven number of divisions to ensure a neutral position. However, some use scales with even divisions to force the respondents to choose an attitude position. Nine-point and

---

Table 4-5 Distortional Use of a Likert Scale

Respondent #1

Item 1	1	2	③	4	5
Item 2	1	2	③	4	5
Item 3	1	2	③	4	5
Item 4	1	2	③	4	5
Item 5	1	2	3	④	5

16 = final score

Respondent #2

Item 1	1	2	3	4	⑤
Item 2	1	2	3	4	⑤
Item 3	1	2	3	4	⑤
Item 4	①	2	3	4	5
Item 5	①	2	3	4	5

17 = final score

11-point scales can be used effectively with well-educated respondents (Warr & Knapper, 1968). The positive and negative poles of the adjectives alternate randomly from one side to the other. This alternation of pairs helps ensure careful reading by respondents.

The attitude object precedes the list of paired adjectives. The attitude object may be a single word, a simple phrase, or a graphic (i.e., picture, design) as indicated in Exhibit 4-1.

Exhibit 4-1 Semantic Differential Scales

Single Word Example

Alcoholic

weak	— : — : — : — : — : — : — :	strong
dirty	— : — : — : — : — : — : — :	clean
valuable	— : — : — : — : — : — : — :	worthless
deep	— : — : — : — : — : — : — :	shallow
tense	— : — : — : — : — : — : — :	relaxed
healthy	— : — : — : — : — : — : — :	sick
bad	— : — : — : — : — : — : — :	good
kind	— : — : — : — : — : — : — :	cruel

Simple Phrase Example

My Clinical Experience

valuable	— : — : — : — : — : — : — :	worthless
deep	— : — : — : — : — : — : — :	shallow
active	— : — : — : — : — : — : — :	passive
tense	— : — : — : — : — : — : — :	relaxed
kind	— : — : — : — : — : — : — :	cruel
happy	— : — : — : — : — : — : — :	sad
ugly	— : — : — : — : — : — : — :	beautiful
fresh	— : — : — : — : — : — : — :	stale

Graphic Example

Graphic

tense	— : — : — : — : — : — : — :	relaxed
quarrelsome	— : — : — : — : — : — : — :	harmonious
pleasant	— : — : — : — : — : — : — :	unpleasant
rejecting	— : — : — : — : — : — : — :	accepting
cold	— : — : — : — : — : — : — :	distant
considerate	— : — : — : — : — : — : — :	inconsiderate
kind	— : — : — : — : — : — : — :	unkind
gloomy	— : — : — : — : — : — : — :	cheerful

Constructing a Semantic Differential

There are five basic steps in constructing a semantic differential: (1) determine the attitude object to be assessed, (2) select appropriate adjective pairs (eight to ten), (3) write complete directions, (4) provide "random polarity," and (5) compute the total score for each respondent.

Early studies by Osgood et al. (1957) used a standard set of ten adjective pairs. Osgood later (1965) expanded these pairs since a major criticism of the semantic differential as a universal instrument was that the same word may not have the same meaning when applied to a different concept. For example, the adjective "heavy" has one specific meaning when it is used to describe a container but a completely different meaning when referring to a young man.

One method of selecting specific adjective pairs to measure a specific attitude concept is to complete an item analysis of the pairs. A manual item analysis procedure is described in the preceding section on Likert scaling. For example, to select adjectives for constructing a semantic differential on attitudes toward the use of nuclear energy it is necessary for the instructor to:

1. Identify two groups of individuals who have pro and anti attitudes toward the use of nuclear energy; it is preferable to use individuals who belong to groups whose specific purpose is known to be opposed or in favor of nuclear power.
2. Ask these groups to use a selection of adjective pairs to describe nuclear power.
3. Complete an item analysis by grouping the results.
4. Use the adjective pairs that best discriminate between the two groups to describe attitudes toward nuclear power; these adjective pairs are said to have "evaluative loadings."
5. Complete the scale using a suitable number of "filler" often unrelated adjective pairs.

The adjective pairs in Exhibit 4-2 with (E) preceding the words have "evaluative loadings" while the pairs preceded by (F) are fillers.

However when adjectives are used to assess all three dimensions of meaning (i.e., evaluative, potency, and activity) the result is improved prediction (Osgood, et al., 1957). Suggested adjective pairs are shown in Exhibit 4-3. The faculty may jointly determine or select the adjective pairs.

The third step in the guidelines, write complete directions, is demonstrated in Exhibit 4-4. The directions there are quite long (as a general rule, they should be as short as possible) but their completeness contributes significantly to the validity and reliability of the results.

Exhibit 4-2 Semantic Differential with Filler Adjectives

(F) pleasant	__ : __ : __ : __ : __ : __ : __ :	unpleasant
(E) harmful	__ : __ : __ : __ : __ : __ : __ :	beneficial
(F) tense	__ : __ : __ : __ : __ : __ : __ :	relaxed
(E) untrustworthy	__ : __ : __ : __ : __ : __ : __ :	trustworthy
(F) gloomy	__ : __ : __ : __ : __ : __ : __ :	cheerful
(E) healthy	__ : __ : __ : __ : __ : __ : __ :	unhealthy

Exhibit 4-3 Suggested Adjective Pairs

good-bad	hot-cold
clean-dirty	angular-rounded
kind-cruel	sharp-dull
happy-sad	optimistic-pessimistic
honest-dishonest	wise-foolish
fair-unfair	believing-skeptical
beautiful-ugly	timely-untimely
rich-poor	dependent-independent
brave-cowardly	large-small
strong-weak	heavy-light
relaxed-tense	sensitive-insensitive
deep-shallow	healthy-unhealthy
thick-thin	cooperative-uncooperative
rugged-delicate	rational-intuitive
active-passive	harmful-beneficial
fast-slow	educated-ignorant

Suggested guidelines for labeling each scale position are shown in Exhibit 4-5. Wells and Smith (1960), in a study of whether scale points should be labeled, report that when eight-point scales are used with or without labels, there are no significant differences in respondents' median scores.

In the fourth step, provide random polarity, adjective pairs should be listed so that positive or negative responses may fall at either end of the scale.

Poor:

good	bad
fair	unfair
friendly	unfriendly
happy	sad
useful	useless

Better:

bad	good
fair	unfair
unfriendly	friendly
happy	sad
useful	useless

Exhibit 4-4 Example of Writing Directions

Directions:
The purpose of this exercise is to assess the *meanings* of certain attitude objects to different individuals. Please make your responses on the basis of what each attitude object means to you. For example, if you feel the concept listed above the adjective pairs is *extremely* related to the high end of the scale, place a check (X) as follows.

relaxed   X : __ : __ : __ : __ : __ : __ : tense

or the low end

relaxed   __ : __ : __ : __ : __ : __ : X : tense

If you consider the concept to be neutral on the scale or if the adjective seems completely unrelated to the concept, place your check (X) in the middle:

safe   __ : __ : __ : X : __ : __ : __ : dangerous

The direction toward which you check depends upon which of the two ends of the scale seems most characteristic of the attitude object.
Please respond with your first impression.

Exhibit 4-5 Guidelines for Scale Position Labeling

Concept

Polar term X __ : __ : __ : __ : __ : __ : __ : Polar term Y

1   2   3   4   5   6   7

1 = extremely X	4 = neither X nor Y	5 = slightly Y
2 = quite X		6 = quite Y
3 = slightly X		7 = extremely Y

Note that the adjective pair may be able to discriminate between two groups when describing attitudes toward nuclear power. However, the same adjective pair may be found to not discriminate when describing attitudes toward abortion. Consequently, depending on the attitude concept to be measured, an adjective pair may be said to have "evaluative loadings" or it may be merely a filler adjective pair.

In the final step, computing the total score for each respondent, an example would involve giving the highest value (7) to the most positive response position, decreasing to (1) for the least positive response position. Since random polarity is suggested, the instructor must be careful to reverse the scoring, as in Exhibit 4-6. The range for the semantic differential scale is 4 through 28. A score of 4 could be interpreted to mean extremely negative attitudes toward women, a score of 28 extremely positive attitudes. Walter's score is 20. While interpretations always are somewhat subjective, it might be concluded that Walter has moderately positive attitudes toward women. If filler adjectives had been used, they would not be included when calculating the final scale score.

Exhibit 4-6 Computation of Total Score

Woman

Useful	(7) : (6) : (5) : (4) : (3) : (2) : (1) : Useless
Dirty	(1) : (2) : (3) : (4) : (5) : (6) : (7) : Clean
Strong	(7) : (6) : (5) : (4) : (3) : (2) : (1) : Weak
Unhealthy	(1) : (2) : (3) : (4) : (5) : (6) : (7) : Healthy

Walter's response to this scale is as follows:

Woman

Useful	__ : __ : X : __ : __ : __ : __ : Useless
	7　6　5　4　3　2　1
Dirty	__ : __ : __ : __ : __ : __ : X : Clean
	1　2　3　4　5　6　7
Strong	__ : __ : __ : __ : X : __ : __ : Weak
	7　6　5　4　3　2　1
Unhealthy	__ : __ : __ : __ : X : __ : __ : Healthy
	1　2　3　4　5　6　7

useful/useless	=	5
dirty/clean	=	7
strong/weak	=	3
unhealthy/healthy	=	5
		20

While the semantic differential often is used to measure attitudes, the score yields only general impressions. It may be particularly useful when the instructor suspects individuals have strong emotional reactions to an attitude object but not a well-developed knowledge base. The semantic differential item can be completed quickly, is not too difficult to construct, and can provide useful information.

As an exercise, students should complete the instructor semantic differential rating form (Exhibit 4-7) for the term "instructor" to determine the warmth rating for the student-teacher relationship.

Exhibit 4-7 Rating Sheet for Instructor Warmth

Directions:
Below are suggested guidelines for each scale position.
Please respond with your first impression as to qualities of your instructor.

Concept

polar term X   — : — : — : — : — : — : — : polar term Y

1   2   3   4   5   6   7

1 = extremely X   4 = neither X nor Y   5 = slightly Y
2 = quite X   6 = quite Y
3 = slightly X   7 = extremely Y

| 1. Cares | 7 : 6 : 5 : 4 : 3 : 2 : 1 : Uncaring |

1. Cares   7 : 6 : 5 : 4 : 3 : 2 : 1 : Uncaring

2. Dislikes   1 : 2 : 3 : 4 : 5 : 6 : 7 : Likes

3. Friendly   7 : 6 : 5 : 4 : 3 : 2 : 1 : Unfriendly

4. Uninterested   1 : 2 : 3 : 4 : 5 : 6 : 7 : Interested

5. Patient   7 : 6 : 5 : 4 : 3 : 2 : 1 : Impatient

6. Accepting   7 : 6 : 5 : 4 : 3 : 2 : 1 : Rejecting

7. Insensitive   1 : 2 : 3 : 4 : 5 : 6 : 7 : Sensitive

8. Nonjudgmental 7 : 6 : 5 : 4 : 3 : 2 : 1 : Judgmental

9. Defensive   1 : 2 : 3 : 4 : 5 : 6 : 7 : Nondefensive

Exhibit 4-7   continued

10. Open	_7_ : _6_ : _5_ : _4_ : _3_ : _2_ : _1_	: Guarded
11. Insincere	_1_ : _2_ : _3_ : _4_ : _5_ : _6_ : _7_	: Sincere
12. Dishonest	_1_ : _2_ : _3_ : _4_ : _5_ : _6_ : _7_	: Honest
13. Untrustworthy	_1_ : _2_ : _3_ : _4_ : _5_ : _6_ : _7_	: Trustworthy
14. Considerate	_7_ : _6_ : _5_ : _4_ : _3_ : _2_ : _1_	: Inconsiderate
15. Harmonious	_7_ : _6_ : _5_ : _4_ : _3_ : _2_ : _1_	: Quarrelsome
16. Supportive	_7_ : _6_ : _5_ : _4_ : _3_ : _2_ : _1_	: Hostile

Amount of Warmth	High 80–112	Moderate 79–49	Low 16–48

Note: Values are listed for purposes of scoring only. They obviously would not appear on the form.

Reliability and Validity of the Semantic Differential

Osgood et al. (1957) cite a number of studies with high test/retest reliability but point out that such a measure is inappropriate since little variability would be expected between the same respondents' rating of the same concept. Warr and Knapper (1968) cite split-half reliabilities ranging from 0.70 to 0.76 for the evaluative subscale, 0.56 to 0.75 for the potency subscale, and 0.58 to 0.66 for the activity subscale. (Split-half reliability is a widely used procedure for estimating reliability. Since practical considerations often require that a reliability estimate be obtained from a single testing, the existing test is divided into two equal halves. A separate score is derived from these equivalent halves. The correlation between these two scores provides a measure of reliability.) Considering the shortness of the scales (i.e., four adjective pairs for each subscale) such correlations are acceptable.

Several attempts have been made to establish predictive and concurrent validity. The purpose of predictive and concurrent validity is to determine the degree of relationship between test performance and other kinds of performance now (concurrent) or in the future (predictive). Positive relationships are reported between semantic differential scales and Thurstone scales (Osgood et al., 1957).

A primary source of invalidity of semantic differential scales is the effect of response bias. Individuals may reply based upon social desirability rather than their true feelings. However, this response bias is a limitation of all assessments of attitudes. Similarly, semantic differential's ability to predict overt behavior is questionable—again, as it also is with other attitude assessment instruments. The semantic differential thus is an acceptable assessment tool for attitude concepts.

THE THURSTONE SCALE

The Thurstone scale, sometimes referred to as an "ordered scale" or "consensual location scaling," was the first method of attitude scaling to be developed (Thurstone, 1931). The Thurstone scale relies upon the evaluation of "experts" whose task is to judge the position of each one of a set of opinion statements on an attitude continuum ranging from "extremely favorable" to "extremely unfavorable." The judges must arrive at a "consensus" regarding the position of each attitude or opinion statement. The final scale provides a weighted score for each item in the instrument. The respondents' own attitudes then are estimated from the weighted scale positions of the items with which they agree.

The model underlying this procedure assumes a probabilistic relationship between attitude position and endorsement of an item. This relationship is represented by the discriminal dispersion for any one item. Discriminal dispersion is a measure of variability that indicates how spread out the data are. The model assumes that these dispersions normally are distributed around a central value representing some point on the attitude continuum (Lemon, 1973). The process of Thurstone scaling involves the ability to determine the discriminal dispersions of a number of items and to select those whose scale values and distributions make them suitable for the final scale.

The discriminal dispersions can be calculated by determining the median position of each statement and the interquartile range for a measure of variability (Lemon, 1973). Quartiles are points on a score scale that divide the area into quarters. The interquartile range is the distance between quartiles. Some researchers recommend calculating the mean position and standard deviation (the measure of variability based on the numerical value of each score in the set of data) of each statement for a measure of variability (Henerson, Morris, & Fitz-Gibbon, 1978).

The statements selected give adequate coverage across the range of scale positions (i.e., 1 through 11) and have a small interquartile range or standard deviation. For example:

> *Poor item statement:* Legal abortions encourage premarital sex.
> Item mean = 3.6
> Item standard deviation = 4.5

Since the standard deviation or degree of spread from the mean is so great, the item should be discarded.

> *Better item statement:* Legal abortions have no effect on premarital sex.
> Item mean = 5.7
> Item standard deviation = 0.57

Since this statement has a smaller standard deviation, it is less ambiguous and should be considered for the final scale.

Once the scale positions are obtained, items are selected carefully for the final scale. These are presented in random order and the scale is ready to be given to respondents.

Constructing a Thurstone Scale

The initial step in constructing a Thurstone scale (Thurstone, 1967) is to determine the attitude variable to be measured.

In the second step, the instructor writes a large number of statements relating to the attitude object that seem to represent a continuum from "extremely negative" to "extremely positive." The statements should be as brief as possible so not to fatigue the respondents reading the list. They should be written so that they can be endorsed or rejected, depending upon the respondents' agreement or disagreement with the attitude being measured. Ambiguous statements should be rejected. Every statement also should be written so that its acceptance or rejection indicates some opinion regarding the attitude. For an example of how not to write it, consider the statement: Nuclear fuel produces electricity. This is merely a statement of fact and as such does not reveal anything regarding respondents' opinions of nuclear fuel.

The instructor then places each edited statement on an item card file, as the third step.

The fourth step involves the instructor's asking a panel of judges, content experts chosen according to the best professional judgment of the individual developing the attitude scale, to sort the items into 11 categories ranging from highly unfavorable (1) to neutral (5–6) to highly favorable (11). The judges should be cautioned that they are making decisions only as to whether the item seems to be valid as it relates to the attitude object; they are not indicating their personal agreement or disagreement with the item. For example, when sorting the statement "I believe in abortion when rape has occurred," the judges should not be asked to agree or disagree but to the best of their ability to give a value as it seems to measure the public attitude toward abortion.

In the fifth step, the items that have been sorted into widely varying categories are discarded. For example, if five judges gave Item 6 the following scale values, it should be considered ambiguous and should be discarded:

Item 6: Sometimes continuing education is a bore.

Item Values by Judge

Judge(s)	1	2	3	4	5
Values	2	3	9	11	8

In contrast, if an item received the following score values it should be considered seriously for the final ordered scale:

Item 7: Continuing education is necessary for all health professionals.

Item Values by Judge

Judges	1	2	3	4	5
Values	11	9	10	9	11

The instructor as the sixth step computes a mean or median value for each score statement. For example, the mean value for Item 7, "Continuing education is necessary for all health professionals," would be 11 + 9 + 10 + 9 + 11 = 50; 50 ÷ 5 = 10.0. Therefore the item's mean value is 10.0; the median also is 10.0.

As the seventh step, the instructor selects a representative sample of 20 to 30 statements so that the completed ordered scale represents items ranging from (1) "highly unfavorable" to (11) "highly favorable."

The assessment instrument then is constructed, in the eighth step, with the order of the statements randomized.

Finally, the instructor records the calculated item scale values for scoring purposes but must not put scale values on the instrument. Exhibit 4-8 is an example for scoring a Thurstone Scale. The statements were written by the author for illustrative purposes only. The score values listed on the right also are only examples; they obviously would not appear on the forms.

Exhibit 4-8 Attitude toward Abortion

Directions:
This is a study of attitudes toward abortion. Below are 20 statements expressing different attitudes.
Put a check (√) mark if you agree with the statement.
Put a cross (X) if you disagree with the statement.
This is not an examination. There are no right or wrong answers. This is simply a survey of attitudes.

Opinion Statements

Student's response		Statement	*Scale Values*
√	1.	It is absolutely immaterial whether abortion is legal or not.	5.5
X	2.	The entire state and national resources should be mobilized to campaign against abortion.	0.4
√	3.	Abortion should be available on a restricted basis.	8.2
√	4.	A ban on abortion is undesirable because it drives women to illegal abortions rather than eliminating it.	9.6
X	5.	Abortion in any form should subject individuals to punishment.	1.0
√	6.	The present proabortion laws are necessary to protect individual rights.	4.2
X	7.	Abortion should be universally permitted.	10.6
X	8.	Abortion laws are desirable now because there is a sufficiently large majority in favor of them.	5.6
√	9.	Both good and bad outcomes have resulted from legalizing abortion.	6.0
√	10.	Abortion prevents many genetic defects and should be encouraged to continue to do so.	6.9
X	11.	The restriction of personal liberty under antiabortion laws is justifiable.	2.9
√	12.	Antiabortion laws are an infringement upon personal liberty.	8.6
√	13.	The effect of abortion on the psychological life of a woman is destructive.	6.0
√	14.	It is every woman's right to decide for herself regarding an abortion.	10.8
X	15.	Abortion is murder.	0.8
X	16.	Laws need to be passed to protect the rights of the unborn.	3.3
X	17.	It is a mortal sin to have an abortion.	0.6
X	18.	Abortion is the only foreseeable way for the world to limit its population.	6.0
X	19.	Abortion is the leading cause of death among babies.	0.9
√	20.	Abortion may help prevent child abuse.	7.0

To calculate the student's overall "pro" attitude or score value, the following formula is used:

$$\text{Score Value} = \frac{\Sigma SU}{N} = \frac{72.8}{10} = 7.28$$

Σ = Sum of

SU = $\sqrt{}$ Score values

N = Number of positive selected statements (those with $\sqrt{}$ before them)

The score value for the student's positive responses is as follows:

5.5	6.0	10.8
8.2	6.9	7.0
9.6	8.6	72.8
4.2	6.0	

When interpreting the attitude scale, it cannot be said that one score is better or worse than another, only that one person's attitude is more pro or con abortion than another person's. For interpreting an attitude scale with 11 divisions, the neutral interval is 5 to 6, the most antiabortion interval is 0 to 1, the most proabortion interval from 10 to 11. The score of 7.28 is slightly above the neutral zone toward fair to moderately proabortion.

Distribution of Attitudes

Figure 4-1 represents a frequency distribution of attitudes toward abortion. A person who is prochoice would be represented to the right of the neutral zone, a person opposed would be to the left. For example, the strength and direction of Ann's score indicate that she strongly favors prochoice. Bob does, too, but more moderately. Eli does not have any strong opinions and Fred is extremely opposed.

It also is possible to compare groups of individuals by a frequency distribution. For example, Figure 4-2 illustrates a hypothetical distribution of males and females regarding attitudes toward abortion. From that graph it could be concluded that most females had definite strongly held attitudes for or against abortion while male respondents were more heterogeneous or spread in their attitudes.

Reliability and Validity of Thurstone Scales

The reliability of the scale can be determined by preparing two parallel forms from the same material and presenting both to the same individual.

Figure 4-1 Distribution of Attitudes toward Abortion

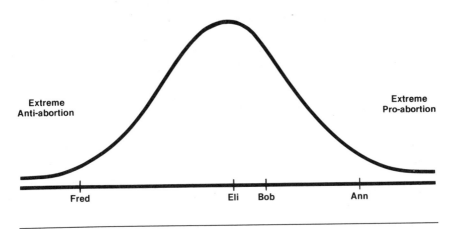

**Extreme
Anti-abortion**

**Extreme
Pro-abortion**

Fred   Eli   Bob   Ann

Parallel forms are equivalent forms of the same material but phrased differently. If the individual has similar scores on both forms the scale is reliable. The correlation coefficient (an index number indicating the degree of relationship between two variables) of the two scores then will indicate the scale's reliability. Since the heterogeneity of the group affects the reliability coefficient, the standard deviation of the score of the group on which the reliability coefficient is determined should be reported. The reliability coefficient is an index number designed to estimate a scale's

Figure 4-2 College Male and Female Opinions on Abortion

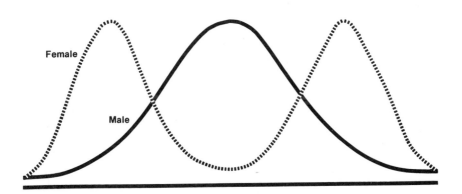

Female

Male

reliability by correlating scores on equivalent forms or scores on two administrations of the same scale. Similarly, the standard error also is an important statistic to be considered when interpreting score results.

If the scale is to be valid, the scale values of the statements should not be affected by the opinions of the individuals who constructed it. For example, an item should be viewed as being in favor of nuclear fuel by either proponents or opponents but not by the tester. When scale values are distorted by the attitudes of the judges, validity is decreased. Hovland and Sherif (1952) report that extremely favorable and extremely unfavorable judges tend to bunch the statements at the opposite end of the scale from their own position. As a result, they give more extreme values than their colleagues who hold less extreme attitudes. This potential decrease in validity can be controlled in part by careful choice of judges and by increasing their number.

The primary limitation of Thurstone scales is that it is difficult to write items that are not ambiguous yet remain unidimensional and extend along a continuum of 11 scale positions.

LIMITATIONS OF ATTITUDE MEASURES

While attitude measures are complex psychological constructs, educators often wish to attempt to measure them. However, when developing and/or interpreting attitude measures, the following limitations should be considered:

• **Inconsistency between measured attitude and behavior:** Neither opinions nor overt acts offer an infallible guide to the assessment of attitude. Much of the research suggests that attitude instruments have relatively weak predictive validity. For example, an individual may score high on a subscale that measures tolerance for differing points of view but in class may denigrate the political views of others. Many variables account for the incongruity between what is said and what is done.

• **Response bias:** If the respondent's attitude measure does not remain anonymous, the respondent may respond in socially accepted ways rather than express true beliefs. Consequently, a climate of acceptance and trust often is a prerequisite for gathering valid data. For example, consider the following item:

I prefer reading to actively participating   SA   A   U   D   SD
in sports.

The individual may really prefer participation in sports to reading but may answer "Strongly Agree" because of the belief that reading is more socially acceptable given the content of the attitude measure.

• **Reliability of the attitude measure:** Fluctuations in the respondent's mood (i.e., illness, fatigue, recent good or bad experiences) all may affect the answer to an attitude measure. Furthermore, if the respondent is not seriously committed to completing the instrument, the reliability will be compromised seriously.

• **Differences in interpretation of the results:** In an instructor-made scale to measure job-related stress that has a possible score range of 15 to 75, Betty may interpret a score of 56 to measure moderate stress and Marie may interpret it as high stress.

• **Adequate time lapse before expecting attitude change:** The factor of time may determine whether the evaluation will emphasize process (i.e., activities, materials) or outcomes (attitudes, values). For example, a four-week summer institute may have the following objective:

The students will increase their sensitivity and respect toward elderly individuals in both community and institutional settings.

However this may or may not be attainable after four weeks of instruction. As a result, the instructor may decide to shift the major emphasis of the evaluation of this objective from outcome to process. For example, did the course materials, activities, and content promote the desired attitude? Did the course include some of the following activities?

• case histories of elderly males and females who hold positions of respect
• selected readings on aging
• volunteer experience with the elderly
• elderly guest seminar leaders.

While this emphasis on process does not negate the necessity of attempting to measure outcomes, it does provide a sound theoretical rationale for process rather than outcome evaluation.

Even though the measurement of attitudes has limitations, many affective behaviors are essential for persons in the helping professions. The development and measurement of these behaviors should be of concern to educators. While educators should not focus on affective behaviors that are not part of the teaching/learning process, they also should not avoid attempting to teach and evaluate other essential affective behaviors.

BEHAVIORAL ORIENTATION ASSESSMENT

Observation is an evaluation technique used frequently for measuring affective behaviors. The observation techniques described in this section vary from highly structured rating scales and checklists to a less structured one—the anecdotal record.

Observation techniques can be used for both formative and summative evaluation. They can be used by (1) faculty observing students, (2) students observing other students (peer assessment), and (3) students observing themselves (self-assessment). The same measurement instrument can be used for all three types of observations.

Observational assessment is a flexible way to collect affective evaluation data. The more observations that can be made with a variety of instruments, the greater the possibility of a valid, reliable assessment.

This section describes the use of three behaviorally oriented assessment instruments: the rating scale, the checklist, and the anecdotal record.

RATING SCALES

Rating scales are widely used observational-based instruments for the measurement of affective objectives. They may include objective information mixed with the instructor's subjective impressions and/or opinions. While rating scales never should be used as the only assessment instrument, they can provide a mechanism for organizing and reporting observations and the instructor's reactions. A rating scale is a selective list of words, phrases, sentences, or paragraphs after which an observer records a "rating" based upon some objective scale of values (Wrightstone, Justman, & Robbins, 1956). Rating scales have two primary components: (1) a set of traits (i.e., stimulus variables) and (2) a scale for each trait indicating the extent to which the student possesses it (i.e., response options).

All educators have had experiences with rating scales. They are rated in elementary and high school, college, and throughout the employment years. Such descriptors as "cooperative," "enthusiastic," "ability to get along with others," and "dependability" are traits often included in rating scales. At times such scales are retrospective (i.e., when a faculty member summarizes impressions developed over an extended period of study) and at other times they are concurrent (i.e., completed after a single encounter, such as after an admissions interview). They are used effectively at times and misused at times. This section analyzes different types of rating scales and variables affecting their validity and reliability and provides suggestions for improving their use.

One of the greatest advantages of the rating scale is its wide range of application, a versatility that makes it extremely useful for assessing affective behaviors. It also is easy to administer and easy to score, can be used with large numbers of students, and can provide important feedback to them regarding their achievement of course objectives.

One of the major disadvantages is not the scale itself but its possible misuse. Faculty members may attempt to assess attributes/variables that are not directly observable. For example, less tangible behaviors such as attitudes toward the elderly are measured more easily by the development of a psychometric attitude scale than by a rating scale.

Numerical Rating Scales

Numerical scales are used to rate traits with numbers that correspond to points on a continuum:

Trait
1. Appearance 1 2 3 4 5
2. Earnestness about nursing as a career 1 2 3 4 5
3. Listening skills 1 2 3 4 5
4. Openness 1 2 3 4 5

Sometimes numerical rating scales have adjective pairs at each end, as in Exhibit 4-9. Ebel (1969) states that the accuracy of a scale is related to its fineness, and the use of large or broad categories is likely to increase the relative amount of error in the measurement.

Exhibit 4-9 Example of a Numerical Rating Scale

Trait					
1. Appearance	1	2	3	4	5
	Sloppy				Well groomed
2. Organization	1	2	3	4	5
	Disorganized				Organized
3. Sensitivity	1	2	3	4	5
	Sensitive				Unsensitive
4. Listening skills	1	2	3	4	5
	Inattentive				Attentive

Graphic Rating Scales

Graphic rating scales frequently are written so that the rater must select some appropriate point in a line instead of choosing a number, letter, or adjective (Thorndike & Hagen, 1969; Wrightstone et al., 1956). A graphic rating scale with directions is illustrated in Exhibit 4-10.

Descriptive Rating Scale

Descriptive rating scales include a more complete description of the set of traits (i.e., stimulus variables) and the response options. A descriptive rating scale is illustrated in Table 4-6. The stimulus variables are not simple words but rather are descriptive phrases that expand upon a stimulus variable. The response options are quantified further by assigning numerical values of 1, 2, 3, and 4 to the descriptive phrases.

Behaviorally Anchored Rating Scales

In Exhibit 4-10, the stimulus variable was expanded to include descriptive phrases; similarly, for behaviorally anchored rating scales, the response options are written in the form of relatively precise behavioral statements. A behaviorally anchored rating scale is illustrated in Table 4-7. Each response option represents a specific point on the scale. The descriptions help increase the rating scale's validity and reliability.

Exhibit 4-10 Example of a Graphic Rating Scale

Directions:

Please place an X along the line in the position that best describes how you feel about the applicant.

Applicant

1. Maturity
   Very Mature   Average   Very Immature

2. Reliability
   Very Unreliable   Average   Very Reliable

3. Dependability
   Very Undependable   Average   Very Dependable

Table 4-6 Example of a Descriptive Rating Scale

Communication Skills	Rare-ly	Occa-sionally	Fre-quently	Consis-tently	Comments
1. Uses professional judgment in selecting, interpreting, and reporting data	1	2	3	4	
2. Communicates effectively with staff and other people	1	2	3	4	
3. Communicates effectively with patients/clients	1	2	3	4	
4. Produces written reports according to requirements of the facility	1	2	3	4	
5. Recognizes and utilizes non-verbal communication	1	2	3	4	

Rank Order Rating Scales

Some rating scales require an individual to rank a number of possible alternatives. It usually is recommended that no more than five items be ranked. The following example illustrates a ranking item:

> Frequently cited criteria for faculty evaluation are listed below. Please indicate, in decreasing order of priority, your ranking of these criteria (1 = most important, 5 = least important).
> Community Service   _____
> Scholarly Productivity   _____
> Personal Growth   _____
> Teaching Effectiveness   _____
> University Service   _____

Rankings made by a number of instructors may be combined into an average rank. The statistical treatment of ranked data is described by Thurstone (1931).

Forced Choice Rating Scales

In the forced choice rating scale, the technique forces the rater to choose between paired alternatives. Both alternatives are favorable but they differ in the extent to which they can discriminate between two groups (i.e., successful and unsuccessful psychiatric nurses).

Example 1:
A. Attends physician rounds periodically to understand patients' status more fully.
B. Experiences success with difficult patients consistently.

Table 4-7 Examples of Behaviorally Anchored Rating Scales

Charts

0	1	2	3	4	5
Not Observed	Unsatisfactory work; poor records of treatment observations.	Charts complete but unorganized; reflect inadequate understanding of patient.	Charts promptly and capably done.	Charts concise; reflect good understanding and follow-up of patient.	Charts are outstanding written record of patient treatment and observations.

Initiative

0	1	2	3	4	5
Not Observed	Not well motivated, unproductive; avoids "doing" whenever possible.	Just getting by; accepts requests but frequently fails to follow through.	Carries share of workload; accepts requests, sometimes volunteers.	Does more than own share of the work; frequently volunteers.	Exceptionally hard worker, conscientious; volunteers, willing to take on extra work.

Example 2:
A. Experiences some degree of success with noncomplaint patients.
B. Establishes contact with hospital psychologist for assistance in understanding problem patients.

Lindeman (1967) reports that the forced choice method of rating scale generally produces more objective and reliable information than other rating scales. However, faculty members often find forced choice items difficult to write. Items need to be written so that they can discriminate yet are similar enough to be appropriate. Properly written items can discriminate between individuals and among skills observed for the same individual.

GUIDELINES FOR CONSTRUCTING SCALES

The initial step in constructing rating scales is to prepare and train raters. Sufficient time and money must be spent on this because, no matter how excellent the rating scale, if it is not administered correctly, the results are invalid. Untrained observers are less likely to obtain agreement than are trained ones. Training sessions should include the philosophy and use of the scale, practice with it, and discussion of the common errors associated with such instruments. During the training, the following additional guidelines will help increase the reliability and validity of the rating procedure (Sinopoli & Block, 1978):

- The evaluation environment should be representative of conditions encountered naturally. For example, an intensive care rotation will expose students to different stresses than will a public health rotation. Therefore, if intensive care is selected for evaluation, all students considered in the same sample should be appraised within ICU. When rotations cannot be uniform, notation of variations should be recorded.
- Sampling of behaviors should be done with care. The decision to use actual/simulated, alert/comatose, cooperative/uncooperative, etc., patients should remain similar throughout the evaluation process.
- Raters should be told how their input fits into the total evaluation plan. The entire plan should be shared with the raters (i.e., clinical instructors). All questions regarding the procedure should be answered before using a specific instrument.
- Raters should be encouraged to vary the number of observations. Drawing inferences from a single incident is not a good sampling procedure. Obviously, behaviors may result from many influences,

which should be reflected in the rating. Generalizations from limited observations are unfair to the student.

The rating form should include a place to note what characteristics were not observed. An item often may be inappropriate, not applicable, or not observable. It also may be desirable to leave space for comments.

In the third step, after the rating scale has been constructed carefully, it should be critiqued and field tested. Academic and clinical faculty members, content experts, and students should review the final draft. The scale should be tested in the actual setting in which it will be used. Final revisions should be made based upon the input from the critiques and that pilot testing.

As the fourth step, the use of specific behaviorally defined anchor points can minimize the inference or judgment that a rater has to make (Exhibit 4-11).

For the fifth step, the instructor should include provisions for three to seven rating positions, which often are recommended for a scale (Dohner, 1974). When assessment requires rough judgments, fewer positions may be required; for finer distinctions, more rating positions. Guilford (1954) suggests that the discriminating power of a scale is lost if it has a small range.

If possible, the sixth step should consist of averaging ratings from several observers to provide a more reliable indicator of student performance. Averaged ratings help eliminate individual rater bias and increase the validity and reliability of the instrument.

As the seventh step, it is essential to identify carefully the specific behaviors to be rated. They should reflect the course objectives. Students

---

Exhibit 4-11 Behaviorally Defined Anchor Points

Poor:					
		Low			High
	Stability:	1	2	3	4
Better:					
	Stability:	1	2	3	4
		Nervous, often panics	Can stand pressure occasionally	Average tolerance for crises, usually calm	Works well under pressure

must be able to identify the link between the classroom objectives and the traits to be measured on the scale. The behavior to be assessed can be complex, such as "establishes a warm, therapeutic relationship with patients." This broad general performance objective must be broken into component parts that represent necessary but not sufficient conditions for effective performance. In Table 4-8, the functional level of warmth is divided into two parts: (1) positive regard and (2) respect. Each of these behavior traits is defined further, as follows:

1. Positive regard: The unconditional acceptance of the patient as a person. Patients are free to be themselves. The students share the patients' hopes and successes as well as depressions and failures.
2. Respect: The students' verbal and nonverbal behavior indicates deep esteem for the patients' problem solving. The students recognize the patients as important to themselves and others.

Exhibit 4-12 offers a scoresheet for rating the levels of warmth under each of the categories in Table 4-8.

Positive regard and respect are included in the rating scale for a functional level of warmth. The descriptors for "degree of warmth" are based on those of Truax and Carkhuff (1967) and Carkhuff (1969).

After these traits are identified in sentence definitions, various levels of achieving them are described. These levels form the fine discrimination illustrated in the rating scale in Table 4-8. It should be noted that this rating scale also includes directions for scoring.

In summary, there should be congruence between the objectives and the rating scale traits; the general performance area should be divided into component parts, with each part described in observable behavior; and the varying levels of achievement should be described.

Grussing, Silzer, and Cyrs (1979) describe the development of a *Behaviorally Anchored Rating Scale* to be used to measure performance of senior pharmacy externs who participate in a 12-week, full-time practicum. They developed a 17-point behaviorally anchored rating scale. The process results in 11 performance dimensions and six personal dimensions on the completed scale. The developed rating scale was used to evaluate extern performance and served as a criterion measure in studies investigating concurrent validity of assessment exercises.

As the final step in constructing rating scales, it is essential not to place similar traits adjacent to each other. Raters tend to give similar ratings to traits in close proximity on a rating form. This produces what is termed proximity error. Consequently, it is recommended that similar traits be placed far apart.

Table 4-8 Rating Scale for Functional Level of Warmth

Positive Regard	Respect

Level 1

Students actively offer patient advice and are indifferent to patient as a person. They often indicate that they know what would be best for patient and are actively critical. Students' overconcern for patient interferes with open and clear discussion.

Level 1

Students' verbal and nonverbal communication conveys a lack of appreciation for patient. Students are more concerned with themselves. In fact they may tell patient more about their own opinions and feelings (i.e., bragging), trying to increase their own self-respect.

Level 2

Students ignore patient, showing little interest or kindness. Students respond passively. Their behavior toward patient varies considerably and is dependent on patient's response.

Level 2

Students' verbal and nonverbal expressions show lack of esteem for patient. However, their interest in and response is dependent on what the patient is talking about. At times students may respond with recognition of patient's worth.

Level 3

Students communicate to patient that patient's feelings and behavior are important to them. Students believe they are responsible for patient and are semipossessive, telling patient, "I want you to. . . ."

Level 3

Students' verbal and nonverbal expressions indicate some degree of appreciation and esteem for patient's feelings and experiences. Students indicate that they value most of patient's opinions and expressions about self.

Level 4

Students show deep commitment, interest, and concern for patient's welfare. They accept patient as a person with little evaluation or criticism of the individual's beliefs or feelings.

Level 4

Students' verbal and nonverbal expressions indicate appreciation for patient's feelings. Their responses enable patient to feel worthwhile.

Level 5

Students show unconditional acceptance of patient as a person. Thus, patient is free to be an individual. Students share patient's hopes and successes as well as depressions and failures.

Level 5

Students' verbal and nonverbal behavior indicates deep esteem for patient's problem solving. Students recognize patient as important to self and others.

Source: Adapted from *Intervention in Human Services* (3rd ed.), by E.D. Schulman, published by The C.V. Mosby Company, St. Louis. Copyright © 1982, by permission of The C.V. Mosby Company. Scale adapted from *Toward Effective Counseling and Psychotherapy* by C.B. Truax and R.R. Carkhuff, published by The Aldine Publishing Company, Chicago, 1967; and *Helping and Human Relations: A Primer for Lay and Professional Helpers* (Vols. I and II) by R.R. Carkhuff, published by Holt, Rinehart, & Winston, New York, 1969.

Exhibit 4-12 Scoresheet for Warmth Scale

Directions:
Place check under one level for each characteristic. The warmth level equals the level
under each category divided by 2 (the total number of categories).

      Example: Positive regard   Level 3
                Respect   Level <u>2</u>
                    Total =   5
              Divided by 2 = 2.5 (level 2+)

			Levels		
Characteristics	1	2	3	4	5
Positive regard					
Respect					
Total number of checks under each category					

VARIABLES AFFECTING VALIDITY, RELIABILITY

Guilford (1954) discusses errors related to rating scale construction and use:

1. Error of leniency: The tendency of the rater to evaluate students' performance higher than actual activity would indicate. This can be avoided in part by the use of precisely stated behavioral response options that help minimize inference and in part by the use of several raters.
2. Error of central tendency: The tendency to cluster all ratings toward the central point, average, or mean. This can be avoided by informing the rater of this danger and by further separating the options that are toward the center of the scale.
3. Halo effect: The tendency to rate students high in all areas because they perform well in a few and are well liked by the rater. The rater does not discriminate among the traits but rather evaluates the students exceptionally high in all. This can be avoided when the rater is assessing several students by rating all on one trait at a time rather than completing the scale on each individual student. This is similar to the suggestions of avoiding the "halo" effect when scoring essay examinations. Essay questions should be scored one at a time.

4. Contrast error: The tendency to rate certain traits in a direction opposite to the rater's own behavior (i.e., raters who believe they are extremely mature may rate all students as immature).
5. Proximity error: The tendency to give similar ratings to traits adjacent on the scale. This can be avoided by using several raters and by rating one trait at a time for all the students and reversing the descriptive adjectives.

Those five errors involve the individual completing the rating scale; however, other errors that are a function of the scale itself can also decrease its validity and reliability. The variables that are not related to the raters but that affect their ability to evaluate accurately are limited observation time and the correctness and/or ambiguity of the trait being measured (Thorndike & Hagen, 1969).

Limited Observation Time

The rater may have limited opportunity to actually observe the student. For example, a clinical instructor who is supervising the clinical experience of 20 students may actually observe each student only three times. Not only may the observation opportunity be limited but the chance to assess such traits as "reaction to criticism" and "initiative" also may be constrained. If the rater has had a limited opportunity to observe the student, the completed rating scales' validity and reliability may be justifiably questioned.

Correctness of Trait Being Measured

Overt aspects of student behavior such as "obtains necessary equipment," "organizes data," "accurately records data," and "neatness" are directly observable and as a result can be rated fairly easily. By contrast, traits such as attitude toward self and others are covert characteristics and are not directly observable. However, just because a trait is not directly observable does not mean that it should be excluded from the rating scale. If the rater has had ample opportunity to observe (and develop some insight into) the individual, the rating of covert traits may provide significant information related to some aspects of the students' social behavior. Furthermore, by increasing the number of overt traits and decreasing the number of covert ones, the scale's validity and reliability will be improved.

Ambiguity of Trait Being Rated

Many rating forms contain traits that are fairly vague and do not have the same meaning for all raters. For example, consider "ability to handle stress." Does it mean a person remains calm in all situations no matter what the stress? Displays self-control compatible with most situations? Becomes upset only in extremely difficult situations?

Improving the reliability and validity of rating scales can be done in a variety of ways, some of them practical, some impractical. To do so, educators should:

- Increase the number of raters. While this is not always practical, it will enhance the reliability of the rating scales.
- Expand description of traits or stimulus variables. The "verbalization" trait can be expanded to "is articulate concerning opinions and ideas" and "has ability to initiate subject matter and ask questions." It also can be replaced by descriptive phrases such as: "verbalizes freely," "takes active role in group discussions," "makes and defends suggestions."
- Expand response categories. A rater often is asked to select a number, letter, or adjective as a response to a stimulus variable. Further refining of the response categories increases the chances that each such category has the same meaning for each rater (see Table 4-9). Educators should be cautioned that there seems to be a critical area between expanding and not expanding the rating scale. Mann (1977)

Table 4-9 Expansion of a Response Category

Self-confidence				
	4	3	2	1
Self-confidence				
	Very High	High	Average	Low
	Adjective Descriptors			
Self-confidence	Displays much confidence. Believes in self and articulates this.	Feels chances of success are good. Believes has ability to initiate projects, ideas, etc.	Feels chances of success are equal to others but needs support.	Feels probability of success is minimal.

reports that when he expanded his interview rating form and made it more descriptive, with the hope of increasing reliability among raters, interviewer complaints concerning the form increased tenfold. In fact, the new form had no significant impact on reliability. Consequently, there seems to be a happy medium that should be striven for when seeking to clarify both traits and response options.

- Rate one trait at a time. This increases the reliability of the rating and helps reduce the halo effect. When each trait is rated simultaneously, the instructor gets an overall impression of the range of behaviors that students elicit in responding to the specific trait. This procedure should be repeated until the entire scale is completed.
- Vary direction of the scale. Rating scales can be written so that positive or negative responses may fall at either end.
- Calculate reliability among raters and for single raters. For interrater reliability, a videotape of a student's performance can be observed by several raters at the same time and their ratings can be compared. For single-rater reliability, the same videotape can be observed by the same evaluator at two separate times and ratings can be compared.
- Couple the rating scale results with anecdotal record reports to document extreme ratings. This linking provides clinical instructors with additional information to verify the "selected" choice. The anecdotal records provide the students with information necessary for changing or continuing behavior patterns. Of course, anecdotal records can document extremely positive behaviors as well as extremely negative ones.

While the validity and reliability of rating scales often are questionable, steps can be taken to enhance their accuracy. However, when the scales are developed carefully and are completed by trained raters who are familiar with the form, they can provide valuable indicators of difficult-to-measure affective traits.

CHECKLISTS: TYPES AND USES

A checklist may be defined as a prepared list of items that may relate to the attitude, value, feeling, or interest being assessed. It may be a list of words, sentences, phrases, or paragraphs describing specific aspects of behavior. The checklist is used for the observation and assessment by which the presence, absence, or frequency of occurrence of each item, phrase, etc., under consideration is checked. In contrast, the rating scale requires a judgment regarding the degree to which a characteristic or behavior is present. Checklists are best used when yes/no kinds of decisions are needed. They frequently are used to evaluate psychomotor skills. They also are being used increasingly to assess interests, attitudes, and personal characteristics.

The checklist offers several advantages for assessing affective behaviors. It (1) is comparatively easy to administer, (2) is easy to score, (3) is low cost, (4) makes feedback interpretation easier, (5) requires only minimal evaluation expertise for effective use, and (6) is extremely objective since the observable outcome is either present or absent.

The primary disadvantage of the checklist is its somewhat limited application. It does not provide a mechanism to qualify or judge the extent to which a behavior or trait is possessed.

When constructing a checklist to evaluate an effective objective, the instructor has a variety of types from which to choose. For example, it may be a "list" of sentences, paragraphs, or words.

Checklist as a List of Sentences

A checklist may be developed that contains a list of sentences. Table 4-10 illustrates a portion of a checklist developed to assess an individual's perception of patient rights.

Table 4-10 A Partial Checklist of Sentences

Directions:
Please respond to the following statements according to the scale below:
   1 = No
   2 = Yes

			Comments
1. The patient has the right to consid- erate and respectful care.	1	2	
2. The patient has the right to refuse treatment to the extent permitted by law and to be told of the medical consequences of the decision.	1	2	
3. The patient has the right to refuse to participate in research.	1	2	
4. The patient has the right to exam- ine and receive an explanation of the bill.	1	2	

Checklist as a List of Paragraphs

Checklists may be developed that contain a list of paragraphs. The example in Table 4-11 illustrates a portion of a checklist developed to assess the leadership potentialities of a relatively new administrator. (In class, the objective is for the students to be able to identify and discuss problems that relate to their new leadership role. The complete checklist appears in Appendix 4-B. It lists some common problems confronted by a new administrator and asks yes/no responses to them. If the respondents answer yes to any common problem, they are directed to discuss it with their direct supervisor. It should be noted that this checklist is made up of paragraphs that describe the specific aspects of behavior to be observed. In this example the checklist is completed not by an observer but rather as a self-assessment.

Checklist as a List of Words

Checklists may contain simply a list of words. Table 4-12 illustrates a portion of a checklist developed to assess the following affective objective: The student will demonstrate a commitment to the improvement of group interaction; when interacting in a group discussion, the student will practice group maintenance functions.

Table 4-11 A Checklist of Paragraphs

| | Does this problem affect you? | | | |
Common Problems	Yes	No	N.A.*	Comment
1. You may feel uneasy. Many factors contribute to a general feeling of uneasiness in a leadership position. Although others have expressed confidence in you, do you have some self-doubt about your ability to do the job?	___	___	___	_____
2. Your job description is generally vague. The higher up in the organization you go, the less specific your job description. More time is spent making decisions than performing specific job-related tasks. Innovation and initiative are expected. Job security may not be available. The workday often extends into the evening. Your performance is more visible to others. Can you deal with this ambiguity?	___	___	___	_____

*N.A. = Not Applicable.

Table 4-12 A Checklist of Words

Maintenance Function	Group Members' Names				
	Edmund	Pauline	Larry	Eileen	Mary
1. Harmonizing		1	1111	1	1111
2. Gatekeeping				1	11
3. Consensus Testing					11
4. Encouraging		1111 1111			11

A complete set of checklists for assessing the affective components of group functioning appears in Appendix 4-C. Because of the importance of the interpersonal side of group functioning and its relationship to the development of interpersonal skills, Appendix 4-C also includes discussions of each checklist.

SUGGESTIONS FOR PREPARING CHECKLISTS

The first step in preparing a checklist is to identify its objectives and determine what specific behaviors are to be observed. Examples of affective objectives that may be assessed by a checklist include the following:

- The student listens attentively when interacting with patients, peers, and faculty.
- The student accepts differences of race and culture.
- The student actively participates in classroom discussion.
- The student demonstrates a commitment to improvement of patient care.

The instructor next involves faculty, students, and/or experts in the development of the checklist. At first glance it may seem that the items will develop automatically from the kind of performance to be observed. However, it is more difficult than it first appears.

For example, when developing a checklist to use as part of a student selection process, views of what are important characteristics to be included may vary from instructor to instructor: What personality characteristics are most important—self-discipline or initiative? What abilities are most important—organizational or communication skills? While the broad line between relevant and irrelevant items is easy to determine, the fine line between the possibly relevant and the possibly irrelevant often is difficult to draw. These decisions often are best determined by the faculty as a whole. Not only should they be accepted by the entire staff, they also should be communicated to the students. In this way the students know that the expectations of all faculty members are similar (Miller, 1962).

If only a representative sample of the faculty is involved in the initial development of the checklist, the rest should be allowed an opportunity to review it and make recommendations for improvements. The involvement of the faculty results in developing a consensus regarding the goals and objectives of the learning activities. This also will strengthen the probability that the checklists will be used as planned, and completed more carefully, resulting in greater validity for the results.

Students also may be involved in checklist development. Another source of items is the expert or board of experts in the specific area or discipline. The best list results from the synthesis of suggestions from a variety of resources (i.e., faculty, students, experts).

The third step is to include an option for nonobserved items. An item may be inappropriate, not applicable, or not observable. If that is true, the form should provide a place to record these nonobservations. In addition, space may be left for comments.

As the fourth step, it is imperative to write clear directions. They contribute to the validity and reliability of the checklist results. Exhibit 4-13 presents an example of clearly written directions.

Exhibit 4-13 Directions for Writing a Checklist

Directions:
Frequently cited reasons for maintaining clinical affiliation agreements are listed below. Please indicate your reason(s) for maintaining agreements by checking the space at the right:
- Required by school administration   _____
- Required by affiliation center administration   _____
- Required to meet eligibility for federal grant funds   _____
- Needed to define duties and obligations of all parties to the agreement   _____
- Needed to prove that the situation exists   _____
- Necessary to provide some assurance of the availability of the
  site for clinical education   _____
- Needed to assist the clinical center with proof of its participation
  in educational activities   _____
- Required to protect the rights of students   _____
- Needed to help assure that all parties are aware of and in
  agreement with the educational objectives of the affiliation   _____
- Other (please specify) _____

The fifth suggestion in preparing checklists is to arrange the items in a logical sequence. Checklists that are written to assess behavior traits may not have any logical sequence. This guideline is especially important for lists that evaluate psychomotor learning.

As the sixth step it is mandatory to prepare the observer adequately. The observer can be anyone who has been taught to use the checklist. The observer should be instructed as to how to recognize the relevant behavior, wait for it to appear, then record it. The better prepared the observer, the more valid and reliable the results from the checklist. As the observer becomes acquainted with the list, the time necessary to complete it will decrease.

Finally, the instructor should test the interpretation of items on a representative sample of observers and students. This will help identify and eliminate vague items. Pilot testing is essential because it will uncover many problems in the phrasing of the items.

CHECKLISTS AND SELF-ASSESSMENT

Checklists often are used for self-assessment. Nursing professionals must be able to evaluate their own behavior objectively because, whether alone or in a team, as professionals they supervise themselves. Therefore they must understand the implications of their actions and accept the consequences of their decisions. They must be able to describe their present abilities accurately and identify areas that need further development.

While self-evaluation skills are necessary, too often little time and effort are spent in the curriculum to develop them. Self-assessment has been found to be valid when compared to (1) test performance (Berdie, 1971; Gilmore, 1973), (2) academic success (Gaier, 1966), (3) peer ratings (Amatora, 1956), and (4) instructor assessment (Geissler, 1973).

Furthermore, self-assessment has resulted in superior work and better critical judgment (Abrams & Kelly, 1974; Geissler, 1973). Individuals experienced with self-assessment techniques tend to be more self-challenging, questioning, analytical, self-motivated, and curious (Wittich & Schuller, 1973).

As a formative evaluation procedure, self-assessment is a powerful and useful strategy. Abrams and Kelly (1974) report the use of a checklist for self-assessment for dental students in cavity preparation. Before using the self-assessment checklist, the students are given lectures and slide demonstrations and are familiarized with the form and the criteria grading components of the course. Abrams and Kelly (1974) report that not only did the self-assessment result in quality clinical performance, it also was effective in promoting a positive attitude toward self-evaluation. Marriner (1974) designed a successful student self-evaluation in a nursing program based on continuous progress toward a previously agreed upon level of performance.

Assisting students in the development of self-assessment may contribute to their accepting the responsibility for their decisions and acts. Today's traditional education system neither teaches nor provides a supportive climate for self-assessment so it must be specifically taught.

Marriner's (1974) research seems to support the idea that self-evaluation has a strong influence on self-esteem and psychological health. Inexperienced individuals often are influenced more by external assessment than by their own self-evaluation. As a result, dependence on external feedback may create a sense of decreased control over their environment. In contrast, individuals with success and experiences in self-assessment can use the external feedback as only one source of information and increase their sense of control over their environment.

Many instructor-centered evaluation instruments such as the checklist can be converted to a self-evaluation format.

VARIABLES AFFECTING VALIDITY, RELIABILITY

To increase the reliability of checklists, (1) instructions should be clear and complete, (2) items should be stated in terms of observable behaviors, (3) the list should not be so long as to fatigue the observer, and (4) there should be a provision for omitting items.

Multiple observations also will increase reliability, as will evaluating students in a familiar setting. Instructors also should share the checklist with the student before it is completed. To enhance the content validity, there must be congruence between the list and the learning objectives.

The checklist is another form of observational assessment. It can complement more traditional types of evaluation procedures. Checklists are relatively easy to use, inexpensive, and can be applied in a variety of clinical and classroom settings. For measuring affective objectives, checklists can evaluate such learning outcomes as teaching effectiveness, communication skills, attitudes, work habits, and interests. They can be developed for use by the instructor (i.e., teacher assessment), for peer assessment, and/or self-assessment.

ANECDOTAL RECORDS

An anecdotal record is a concise and objective written report, based on direct observation, describing an incident in an individual's behavior

(Thorndike & Hagen, 1969). In more general terms, anecdotal records are a series of brief descriptions of behavior. As successive observations accumulate, the record becomes a more valid and reliable indicator of the student's interests and attitudes. The accurate recording of behavior in anecdotal records provides objective descriptions of individuals in their relationship with each other and their environment.

Well-written anecdotal records can:

1. provide instructors with insights to understanding the behavior of their students that may aid in fostering their personal/social development
2. provide information that can be used with other types of assessment to evaluate affective educational objectives (i.e., personal, social, and emotional adjustment, and growth).

Exhibit 4-14 is an example of a typical anecdotal record form. Single observations may be recorded on file cards—three inch by five inch or five inch by eight inch.

ADVANTAGES AND LIMITATIONS OF DATA

Ancedotal records can provide an informal and qualitative picture of students' behavior that is unavailable from more traditional sources of

---

Exhibit 4-14 Example of an Anecdotal Record Form

```
            Name of School: _____

            Anecdotal Record: _____

Date: _____ Name of Student: _____

                         Class: _____

Setting:


Description of Incident:


Comment/Interpretation:



                    Observer's Signature _____

                           Date _____
```

information. By observing students interacting with others in either natural and/or simulated situations, the instructor can gain information beyond more easily measured cognitive information.

The primary limitation of this type of data is observer bias. Each observer may perceive an event differently. This "selective perception" and/or "selective retention" may affect how individuals describe and interpret events. The validity of the observations thus is dependent upon the objectivity of the observers.

Two persons who witness the same event can assign to it different meanings that may be the result of a series of complex factors such as previous experiences, expectations, needs, desires, and values. Observers' perceptions of events affect their subsequent written anecdotal records. Perception is affected by values, beliefs, self-concept, communication skill, knowledge, and the context in which the events occur. Context includes the physical setting, persons involved, time, and cultural influences. Finally, perception can be affected by "noise," defined in this context as anything that interferes with accurate interpretation of the event. For example, noise can be physical (horns honking, babies crying, telephones ringing) or psychological (feelings, values, prejudices). Consequently, different observers will record varying views of the same actual observed event.

Each faculty member recording an event adds an interpretation—perhaps the same as the source intended, perhaps not. Observers also perceive differently because of variances in their environmental and experiential backgrounds. The realization and acceptance of that fact can improve communication.

Selective Perception

Perception is how each person sees the world. It involves all of the senses: seeing, hearing, smelling, tasting, and touching. It is different for each individual. How people perceive the world is dependent upon their own personal life experiences. For example:

- Paul may smell suntan lotion and immediately remember the lazy summer days at the ocean; in contrast, Janice may recall painful sunburn.
- John may see a picture of the ocean and immediately remember the summers of his youth where he vacationed with his family; Kelly may see the ocean and her pulse may rise because of her fear of the water because she saw her brother drown when she was 4 years old.

- Elizabeth may hear classical music and remember her childhood because, for the first 17 years of her life she was awakened at 6:30 a.m. by her father's favorite radio station playing classical music; Elaine may recall a childhood cartoon television show that always used classical music as background.
- Paul may taste chicken curry and remember Claudette, a Guyanan friend who first introduced that flavor to him; Mike may spit it out immediately because of its hot taste.
- Deane may be touched by a male friend and the contact may make them closer; Debra may be touched by a male friend and instantly feel repulsion because it reminds her of the frequent sexual attacks by her stepfather when she was 13.

So while everyone perceives through the senses, each individual sees, hears, smells, tastes, and is touched differently. Because of this, they see, interpret, and record events differently. This effect of "selective perception" should be kept in mind in recording and interpreting anecdotal records.

Selective Retention

As individuals selectively perceive information, they also selectively retain it. For example, a person especially fond of John will selectively remember most of his strengths; in contrast, a person who is not particularly fond of him may recall only his weaknesses. This is called "selective retention."

As instructors prepare anecdotal records they should keep in mind that the validity of their observations is affected by "selective perception" and "selective retention." Just as people are selective in what they perceive, so also are they in what they choose to remember.

Selective perception and selective retention may become obstacles when recording information for an anecdotal record.

Time and Skill Factors

Another limitation of anecdotal records is that they are very time consuming to write. Instructors often do not have the time to prepare, summarize, and file the records.

Finally, good anecdotal records require a skilled observer who can describe behavior sequentially and nonjudgmentally. This requires practice and training.

All information on anecdotal records should be interpreted cautiously. It must be remembered that the data collected are intended to contribute to the social growth of the students.

It is this author's firm belief that all anecdotal records should be destroyed at the end of each semester and that they never should become a part of the student's permanent record. The problems of sampling error, selective perception, selective retention, and ultimate rater bias are too great to suggest that they become a part of the permanent record.

GUIDELINES FOR ANECDOTAL RECORDING

A number of specific steps serve as a guideline for preparing anecdotal records (Wrightstone, Justman, & Robbins, 1956). The first is that each entry must be dated. This makes clear the sequence of anecdotal events when the record is reviewed. That sequence may be crucial to the interpretation of the data.

The second requirement is that observations be recorded on the day they occur. That way they are less likely to be distorted by dimming memory. The longer the delay between the observation and the recording of the event, the less valid the report.

In the third step, each entry should be preceded by a statement that describes the setting in which the incident occurred. For example, a student breaking into tears before an examination is quite different from one crying after observing a stillborn delivery.

As the fourth step, each entry should contain a brief factual description of the incident. While the emphasis is on listing factual information, ease of recording, rather than grammatical excellence, is desirable. A sample entry:

> Jan. 10, 1983, 10:15 a.m.: John fell asleep during class. He awoke when spoken to, was attentive for a few moments, then fell asleep again.

There are a number of common errors to avoid when recording factual information. For example, reporting generalizations rather than specifics:

Examples of generalizations:
- Talks all the time.
- Is lazy.

Examples of specifics:
- Interrupted his peers six times during a ten-minute discussion.
- Turned in all three assignments late.

For another example, reporting personal reaction rather than observed behavior:

Personal reaction:
  • Susan is a thoughtful, considerate student.

Observed behavior:
  • Susan volunteered to tutor Alpedia, a new foreign student.

The fifth step calls for separating the factual description of an incident from the interpretation of it. For example:

Poor: Jason repeatedly showed his hostility to the "prolife" speaker by firing questions at her throughout the presentation. His constant interruptions were bothersome to many of his peers. He was asked to "please, be quiet" many times. It was apparent that Jason was proabortion and unwilling to consider other points of view.
Better:
Setting: Prolife presentation
Incident: Jason fired questions throughout the presentation. He persisted even when the speaker suggested that there would be time for questions at the end of her presentation. Three times his peers asked him to be quiet.
Comment: Jason seemed to be unwilling to consider another point of view.

The sixth step is that the observer must document both positive and negative events. It is just as important to record events that illustrate exemplary behavior as it is the less desirable. This provides a more complete, unbiased record. Some observers document only negative events, thus providing a distorted view of the performance.

As the seventh step, it is necessary to document a number of observations per student before drawing inferences regarding behavior. An adequate number and sequence of events will increase the reliability and validity of the records. The observer should try to record at least one entry per week per student. For example:

September 7. Maria refused to feed Mr. Charles, a stroke patient, and asked to help pass medications instead.
Comment: Maybe she doesn't have the patience to feed an adult patient.
September 14. Maria again refused to help Mr. Charles feed himself even though he seemed to be improving. Maria asked to be assigned to Mr. Baron, a young burn patient. She took time and care feeding Mr. Baron and changing his dressings.
Comment: Maria does seem to have patience, possibly a deliberate attempt to avoid Mr. Charles. Very unusual behavior for Maria.
September 21. Maria refused to help Mr. Charles with his walker and ran out of his room in tears.
Comment: Upon questioning, Maria revealed that she was helping care for her father, who had had a cerebrovascular accident with right hemiplegia. She and

her mother had been caring for him for three years. Mr. Charles reminded her of her father and she couldn't help care for him.

By recording a series of events, a better understanding of Maria's behavior was obtained. Generalizations should be arrived at only after several independent observations; even then, they should be done conscientiously and cautiously. It is a common error for observers to interpret data before they have an adequate number of observations.

In the eighth step, the observer should practice writing anecdotal records. At first the instructor may find this difficult and time consuming. However, with practice the task does become easier. The instructor should begin by writing anecdotal records for only a few students and, if they seem to be yielding useful information, expand to include more students. It should be remembered that the goal is brevity and clarity, not literary style.

In the final step, the instructor should learn to limit each record to a description of a single event. For example:

> *Poor:* Martha was preparing Miss D.E. for a saline abortion. It is suspected that Miss D.E. has been impregnated by an older brother. Martha exhibited the most empathetic listening responses when caring for the patient. However, yesterday Martha was preparing Mrs. L.R. for a dilation and curettage. Mrs. L.R., the wife of a prominent local businessman, has two children, and does not want another. While preparing Mrs. L.R., Martha's responses were sharp, rude, and insensitive.
>
> *Better:*
> *Setting:* Clinical Rotation in OB
> *Incident No. 1:* Martha was preparing Miss D.E., age 15, for a saline abortion. It is suspected that Miss D.E. has been impregnated by an older brother. Miss D.E. told Martha, "I just feel bad inside, that's all. Do people ever really consider killing themselves?" Martha responded, "I hear you saying that you're feeling pretty hopeless today."
> *Comment:* Martha's response recognized and reflected Miss D.E.'s feelings.
>
> *Incident No. 2:* Martha was preparing Mrs. L.R. for a D & C. Mrs. L.R., the wife of a prominent businessman, has two teenagers, and does not want another child. Mrs. L.R. told Martha, "Last week I walked out of the hospital, unaborted, but here I am again." Martha responded, "You should have stayed home."
> *Comment:* Martha's response still did not recognize and reflect Mrs. L.R.'s feelings.

VARIABLES AFFECTING VALIDITY, RELIABILITY

There are several sources of reliability errors for the anecdotal record:

- the emotional/physical well-being of the observer may influence judgment as to which observational data to record

- the observation skills among instructors may vary
- the instructors' preferences, expectations, needs, feelings, and personal biases may distort their observations.

A limited number of written observations can decrease the content validity of anecdotal records.

COUNSELING ORIENTATION

This section describes the counseling approach to the assessment of affective objectives. The counseling interview is an excellent way for faculty and students to mutually explore perceptions and values that influence behavior. Interviewing involves a complex interaction and synthesis of factors such as questioning and communication skills, ability to infer meanings and respond accordingly, and knowledge of attitude development and formation.

Three levels of interviews and their relationship with the counseling approach are:

1. the information-oriented interview
2. the experiential interview
3. the behavior modification interview.

Instructors become involved in all three, whether or not they are adequately trained and/or prepared.

THE INFORMATION-ORIENTED INTERVIEW

The information-oriented interview's primary purpose is to gather data regarding people, events, programs, places, etc. The instructor seeks facts and/or opinions about some predetermined objective. For example, the nursing faculty may be involved in selecting students for an obstetric internship:

Interview objective: To select the best candidate for a nurse practitioner internship in obstetrics.
Information to be obtained:
  1. the student's general perceptions regarding obstetric nursing
  2. the role of the nurse in the delivery and administration of nursing care
  3. the student's general knowledge of obstetric nursing
  4. the student's personal concerns as they relate to the rotation.

Exhibit 4-15 is an example of an interview questionnaire that may be used as a guide for gathering information from a prospective student.

The information-oriented interview may use a structured or an unstructured format. In the structured interview (as in Exhibit 4-15), the wording and sequence of questions are predetermined. In contrast, in the unstructured format, key questions about the topic of interest are asked but the basic approach is nondirective, providing an opportunity to explore spontaneous responses.

The following dialogue illustrates a directed interview. The dialogue is between a nursing faculty member and a prospective student for the obstetric unit. It should be noted that the directed interview is a fairly thorough and concise method of gathering information.

Norma: What do you believe to be your strongest and weakest points?

Diana: Well, that's difficult to answer without some thinking time. I guess my strongest assets are that I'm hardworking and that I thrive on challenges. For example, I didn't go to nursing school until after my third child was born, but once I started I maintained respectable grades and was responsible for most of the care of the children because my husband was in Vietnam. However, my mother did help a lot.

My weakest point I guess is my impatience. Change is so slow and waiting for new ideas to be implemented is so frustrating. For example, during my pediatric internship in a small rural hospital they were still giving alcohol rubs to infants with high fevers. I tried to explain that the alcohol was readily absorbed and that it was not a recommended procedure. However, they said it was "routine procedure" and refused to read some current research on nursing care for children with high fevers. It was so frustrating for me.

Norma: How important do you believe a sense of humor is to your work?

Diana: Very important. Working in a hospital, people are often under a great deal of stress, both the personnel and the patients. Humor often helps reduce the stress.

Norma: What qualities do you believe a good clinical instructor should possess?

Diana: Interpersonal skills are most important. Clinical instructors need to be able to communicate with their students verbally and in writing. I don't mind being told that my charting notes need to be improved if I'm also offered some suggestions for improvement.

Norma: If you were chosen for this internship what three things would concern you most?

Diana: Well, first I would like the opportunity to learn and grow professionally. I would like as many different challenges as possible. Secondly, it would be nice to know that my suggestions and/or concerns would be seriously considered. And finally I would like to successfully complete the rotation.

In this directed interview the instructor really does "direct" the session by following a rather rigid outline to glean the information needed. The

Exhibit 4-15 Example of an Interview Questionnaire

1. *General Perceptions*

   - How would you describe the essential personality attributes of a good obstetric nurse?
   - How do you distinguish between nursing care for the normal full-term pregnancy patient and the abortion patient?
   - What role do you feel you could play in a patient education program?
   - What models of nursing care plans are you aware of? How may these models be relevant to this institution?

2. *Nurse Role*

   - What criteria should be used to identify the best nurses for an obstetric nursing position?
   - Can you identify some nurses who meet those criteria?
   - How would you facilitate the change from functional nursing to primary care nursing?
   - Would you help to promote the establishment of a better patient education program?
   - What incentive systems could be established to encourage departmental participation in a patient education program?

3. *Content*

   - How would you describe nursing care for a patient with placenta previa with toxemia and with diabetes mellitus?
   - How would you contrast the nursing care of a patient who has had a saline injection abortion and one who had an abortion by dilation and curettage?
   - What are the major components of childbirth classes?

4. *Personal Concerns*

   - What do you believe to be your strongest and weakest points?
   - What motivates you to put forth your greatest efforts?
   - What are your short-term and long-term goals?
   - What qualities do you believe a good clinical instructor should possess?
   - What three things would concern you most if you were chosen for this rotation?
   - How do you believe a student's worth should be judged?

results can be used to gather information needed about a potential student that could not be gleaned from a transcript of grades from previous educational experiences.

INFORMATION-ORIENTED INTERVIEW GUIDELINES

The first step in constructing an information-interview is to identify its purpose and objectives. Interviews may be used to accomplish many objectives, such as:

- an admissions interview
- an assessment of the integration of clinical and didactic knowledge
- assistance in the diagnosing of student performance problems.

Next, it must be determined whether the interview will be structured or unstructured. The structured interview includes predetermined questions and often requires simple direct responses; the unstructured form can be compared to a conversation between two people.

Either type of interview may contain closed or open-ended questions. Closed questions restrict the student's response to a brief answer. For example, "What is the average number of hours you spend in the clinic per week?" Open-ended questions allow a greater expression of feelings, provide for an unlimited range of possible answers, and may result in providing feedback for constructing important closed questions for future interviews.

In the third step, the instructor drafts and critiques the questions. Following are guidelines for critiquing questions. The instructor should:

1. Include only one idea per question:

   Poor: Are students invited to share their knowledge and experiences and to criticize the instructor's own ideas?
   Better: Does the instructor invite students to share their knowledge and experiences? Are students invited to criticize the instructor's own ideas?

2. Write simple, short, direct questions:

   Poor: According to your observations, the data from the chart, and the laboratory findings, is this child experiencing cardiac duress?
   Better: Is the child experiencing cardiac duress?

3. Avoid questions that may evoke negative emotional responses:

Poor: Do you need considerable supervision in the intensive care unit?
Better: What amount of supervision do you consider "ideal" for you in the intensive care unit?

4. Avoid "loaded" questions that encourage one answer and discourage another:

Poor: Is your coworker a malingerer?
Better: How much initiative does your coworker exhibit?

As the fourth step, the instructor should provide adequate introductory information to the interview:

Poor: This interview will be used to provide us with data regarding your internship.
Better:

Describing purpose	This interview will be used to provide us with some data regarding your internship in the coronary care unit.
Describing how the information will be used	The information will be used as part of your application, along with letters of recommendation.
Role of interviewer	I will be completing the interview and will be responsible for summarizing the information for the review by the admissions committee.

Adequate introductory information is as essential as adequate directions are for a questionnaire. It increases the relative reliability and validity of the information. In the better example, the instructor stated the purpose of the interview, explained how the information would be used, and described the instructor's role in the process.

Pretesting of the interview constitutes the fifth stage. The pilot testing will help identify problems such as inconsistency in logic and/or sequencing of questions and will identify complex, negative, and/or "loaded" questions.

Instructors will have greater success if they have some experience with using the instrument (i.e., structured or unstructured interview) and some basic knowledge of listening and counseling skills. An integration of these skills with the interview is likely to provide the anticipated information.

The sixth and final step is for the instructor to record all comments regarding the interview immediately. In summarizing reactions, it is vital not to trust memory. If the recording of comments is delayed, a great amount of potentially valuable information may be lost.

THE EXPERIENTIAL INTERVIEW

The experiential interview features the sharing and understanding that enter into experience, with the students' personal growth as the primary purpose. While the experiential interview may contain some information-oriented questions, these serve only as secondary information. This type of interview stresses the empathetic interaction between instructor and students. It often takes place during a crisis in the students' life or when the instructor is assisting them in developing insight into their own behavior and personality.

This type of interview is extremely important in the everyday life of an instructor. The following example is a brief introduction to an experiential interview:

Instructor:	Hi, please sit down. Excuse the mess, I'm preparing for report.
Sue:	Do you care if I smoke? I stopped but I've started again. Too nervous. I don't know where to begin. Can't talk to anyone, not my parents, not my best friend, not John.
Instructor:	Hmm. You seem anxious. Need someone to listen. I'm here.
Sue:	I'm pregnant.

So begins the experiential interview. The closer the interpersonal relationship between the instructor and the student and the longer the student has been at the hospital, the more likely the instructor will be actively involved in experiential interviews. Obviously, they require an unstructured format.

In the experiential interview, as noted, the instructor and the student share feelings, understandings, and behavior. For example:

Ellen:	(Enters the instructor's office and sits in the chair opposite Ms. L.)
Ms. L:	(Looks up from her work and smiles.)
	Hello, Ellen. Nice to see you on this warm fall day.
Ellen:	(Staring at her reports.)
	I can't get my reports finished by Friday, too much work to do. Everything is due at once.
Ms. L:	Yes, I remember how hectic the end of the semester always was. But your outline and first draft were excellent. It should be relatively easy for you to complete it after all your work on the first draft.

Ellen: (Still staring at the wall.)
I just can't concentrate. Nothing much seems to matter any more—What's the use? In the end we all die.

Ms. L: You seem to be telling me you are depressed.

Ellen: My mother called last night. Dad left and wants a divorce.

Ms. L: (Silent)

Ellen: A divorce! After 24 years of marriage! I know their life has not always been happy but no one was ever guaranteed happiness. Mom wants me to come home for the weekend. She needs someone to talk to. How can I help her? I feel like someone just died.

Ms. L: Yes, I know, divorce is somewhat like death. It marks the end of a relationship.

Ellen: But Mom doesn't want the divorce. She was crying hysterically over the phone. What can I do? I can't make Dad come home. How can I help?

Ms. L: Would it help your mother to see you this weekend?

Ellen: Yes, I guess . . . but I'm not sure I can be of any help. Maybe if I was just "there," maybe just being there would help.

Ms. L: Sometimes it just helps to have someone near to share the grief.

Ellen: My damn, damn, damn father! Do you mind if I'm not in class on Friday?

For this kind of experiential interview to take place, the instructor probably has created an accepting climate already. The instructor has demonstrated respect for the students and a genuine interest in their welfare. The instructor thus has created an environment that promotes complete confidentiality. It should be noted that the instructor asked relatively few questions and did not offer any "solutions" to Ellen's problem but rather was an active listener.

The experiential interview also can be useful when routine faculty observations uncover possible behavior problems. These should be regarded as general impressions since the behavior may have multiple interpretations. For example, suppose Heather received an evaluation on listening skills like that shown in Exhibit 4-16. The instructor asks her to come in to discuss the evaluation.

Heather: I don't think it's fair. I listen carefully most of the time.

Instructor: I hear you saying you listen most of the time. Can you share instances when you didn't listen?

Heather: Women in labor bug me. I can't understand why they have to carry on and yell so much. You know it gets hectic in the labor room and sometimes it's impossible to meet everybody's demands.

Instructor: You were very kind to Mrs. Calhoun, yet she was in labor.

Heather: Yeah, but she was fairly quiet and didn't yell or scream.

Instructor: Take a minute and write down the names of all the patients you have cared for in the delivery room this week. Then score each one according to how much you enjoyed caring for them.

Heather: (Writes the list)
Wow, it looks like I enjoy caring for the quiet ones.

Exhibit 4-16 Evaluation of Listening Skills

____	____	_X_
Displays outstanding attending behavior	Generally displays attending behavior	Often ignores questions and comments

The experiential interview provides instructor and student with a way to identify problems, consider alternative explanations, and select solutions. However, both must be willing to explore the problem behavior mutually. The instructor also must communicate that the problem is understood and that the student is respected. When this is done, the student can develop a sense of optimism about solving the situation.

There may be times when there are differences of opinion about the existence of a problem. These may involve differences of perception or of values (Gordon, 1978). Perception differences are disagreements about what is true. They often can be resolved by collecting data to determine who is right.

For example, an instructor believes a student is insensitive to others' value systems. To resolve the perception differences, custom-designed checklists or anecdotal records may be useful. Three key steps of problem assessment should be taken: (1) identifying relevant behaviors mutually, (2) collecting data, and (3) analyzing the data together. The most important variable is: Are the data of sufficient quantity and quality to be credible to the student and the faculty member? Value differences are disagreements about what is important; they do not yield to empirical evidence.

> *Instructor:*   Your uniform is often disorderly and untidy and your shoes are rarely clean.
>
> *Heather:*   I know, but a tidy uniform isn't important. What's important is the quality of the nursing care I give.

An examination of value differences may modify positions, at the very least, it creates a better understanding of the opinions held. While affective and communication skills are useful for all types of counseling, they are especially crucial to the experiential interview.

AFFECTIVE SKILLS

The affective skills of expressing empathy, demonstrating positive regard, and developing trust can greatly improve the effectiveness of any kind of interview. They are briefly described next.

Expressing Empathy

Empathy is the feeling and sharing of other persons' feelings about their experiences (Schulman, 1982). Its general characteristics are unconditional acceptance accompanied by an openness to considering different value systems, accurate processing of information, and concrete feedback.

- Unconditional Acceptance: This is built upon openness as reflected in genuineness and warmth. A prerequisite to unconditional acceptance of others is self-acceptance.

- Openness to Different Value Systems: Openness to different attitudes and values will assist the instructor in obtaining the necessary information accurately. It is easier to gain more information and to recognize gaps in what has been presented. Openness decreases the errors inherent in selective perception. Selective perception occurs when instructors see and hear only what they "want" to hear. For example, a student may come to class late and be physically unkempt. An open instructor may suggest a private meeting to determine the reasons for the tardiness. In contrast, a closed-minded instructor may merely record an unsatisfactory.

- Accurate Processing of Information: This is essential during an interview. The ability to glean relevant information and to record changes in mood accurately help increase the validity of the interview.

- Concrete Feedback: During the interview, concrete intermittent feedback increases the likelihood of more responses from the interviewee.

An example of concrete feedback in operation:

Student: I must talk to you about quitting school. I don't think I can handle it anymore. I was up all night crying.

Instructor: You seem to be upset. Are you upset about school?

Student: Well, that's part of it, all the assignments and with finals starting I don't think I can get everything done. Anyway, it's not important to me. Dan, my husband, told me he's not sure he loves me anymore. I've always been so sure of his love. Now that he's not sure, all I do is cry. He tells me not to cry, not to keep asking him why, but I can't. I can't do anything. All I want to do is to sit-sit-sit! I didn't even go out of the house last weekend.

Instructor: I'm hearing something else now. School doesn't seem to be the real problem.

Instructors' unconditional acceptance of students, their openness to different attitudes and values, their accurate processing of information, and their ability to give valued concrete feedback will help make interviews an effective tool for assessing the affective domain.

Demonstrating Positive Regard

An individual expressing positive regard exemplifies the degree of positive feelings one person has for another. No experience should be considered unworthy of positive regard. As a result, the instructor remains open and understanding, regardless of what the student wishes to discuss.

It does not matter whether the experience is socially unacceptable. The student is valued because of who the person is, not because of experiences, attitudes, or values. Positive regard does not mean agreement or approval; it merely means respect or liking.

Developing Trust

Obviously, trust cannot be developed during an interview; only the beginning of sowing the seeds for trust can be made. The instructor at least can try to begin the interview by establishing rapport with the student.

The rating scale in Appendix 4-D illustrates a way to measure the instructor's functional level of empathy. It could be used as a self-assessment tool for the instructor to answer the question: "During the experiential interview, was I empathetic?" It also could be modified slightly to determine a student's functional level of empathy.

COMMUNICATION SKILLS

In addition to the affective abilities of expressing empathy and positive regard, and developing trust, a number of communication skills can facilitate interviewing techniques. They include attending behavior, paraphrasing, reflecting feelings, summarizing content, and providing assistance.

Attending Behavior

When instructors exhibit "attending behavior," they notice the student's verbal as well as nonverbal behavior. For example, is the student's posture stiff and rigid? Are the arms opened or crossed? Are the feet, hands, or legs in constant motion?

For example, the nonverbal behavior that seems to indicate acceptance is a relaxed body posture conveyed by slightly leaning forward or sitting forward in a chair, and loose, natural arm, hand, and leg movement, with eye contact.

Mehrabian (1972) suggests that threat and anxiety are noted through changing the subject. Physical proximity, leaning forward, and direct eye contact reveal positive feelings. Relaxed posture and position also often reveal positiveness and status. As a result, individuals with higher status tend to be more relaxed.

Facial and body clues also are important to observe during interviews. Kendon (1972) reports that duration of gaze indicates a more positive relationship. Consequently an individual wishing to convey intimacy will give a direct, relatively prolonged gaze.

Ekman and Friesen (1969), in a study of facial expressions and hand and leg gestures as they relate to honesty, find that when individuals are communicating honestly, they show greater foot and leg movement than when they are being dishonest. Effective interviewers not only observe nonverbal behavior but also stop to listen. They are not preoccupied with their own thoughts.

Paraphrasing

Paraphrasing is a form of restating or translating. The listener rewords the statement and repeats all the important points. The purpose is to enhance the understanding by concentrating on ideas.

> *Student:*   I don't seem to be able to make friends, I'm lonely. I even went to the movies alone last night. Maybe it's because I'm black.
> *Instructor:*   Hmmmm. A case of loneliness.

Reflecting Feelings

A statement in fresh words is useful in expressing the students' essential attitudes and feelings. The instructor must withhold judgment. Reflection of feeling is not an end in itself but rather a means of assisting the students to see the dimensions of the problem. It is hoped that this new insight will enable the students to reorganize their thinking and to seek appropriate solutions.

Adequate reflection of feeling assures the students that the instructor understands what is being said. In practice, accurate reflection of feeling is difficult and depends upon the affective skills of listening and empathy. The students are told that the instructor understands not only what is being said but also what is being felt. For example:

> *Diane:*   All I keep thinking is "Woman, you missed the boat again! You got the dream but not the brains."
> *Instructor:*   I hear you saying that you feel discouraged.

During reflection of feeling, the feelings typically are classified as positive, negative, or ambivalent. In the course of a good interview, feelings are likely to change from negative to ambivalent to positive (Exhibit 4-17).

In practice, reflection of feeling is not learned easily because it runs contrary to people's long experience of responding primarily to content. In the beginning it may be useful to vary introductory phrases such as:

"I hear you saying that . . ."
"As I understand . . ."
"In other words . . ."
"It seems to me that . . ."
"I gather you believe that . . ."
"You seem to feel that . . ."

While it is important to reflect what has been heard, the instructor also should reflect nonverbal behaviors. Frequently gestures, posture, and/or tone of voice express something the student has not yet been able to verbalize:

"You look sad . . ."
"It seems difficult for you to discuss this . . ."
"You seem anxious . . ."

If the instructor inaccurately reflects nonverbal behavior, the students have the opportunity to deny the teacher's interpretation. However, such reflections may assist the students in better understanding their feelings.

Summarizing Content

While summarizing content somewhat overlaps with paraphrasing, the primary difference is the amount of information covered. In this mode, the instructor tries to summarize the totality of the ideas and feelings that were expressed during the interview.

Joanna: I have a problem getting to work on time. Oh, I can do it, but finding the time to come with polished shoes and a pressed uniform is

---

Exhibit 4-17 Reflection of Feeling

The instructor comments:		
___ Negative	___ Ambivalent	___ Positive
"You really are upset about your clinical evaluation results."	"Even though you are upset, you feel in some ways you are making progress."	"You are going to continue working hard. With help, you can make it."

difficult. And then there's the kids. I have to clean up after them
over and over! I don't think I've had time for myself since I began
school. I had a bloody nose last night and I think my blood pressure
is up. My father died of a stroke. I'm tired of it all. . . .

Instructor: I gather that you're pretty frustrated coping with work and home.
That's what I hear you saying. I understand. And you are worried
about your health.

The instructor should avoid communicating a note of finality at the end
of the interview. It also is important during summarizing content to communicate the fact that the instructor understands the student's point of
view. When students believe they are understood, (1) they feel and perform
better, (2) their level of anxiety is reduced and (3) the understanding implies
acceptance (Bernstein, Bernstein, & Dana, 1974). While acceptance does
not imply approval or agreement, it does indicate that the student is valued.

The Scale for Rating Communication Skills illustrated in Chapter 3 can
be used to determine a functional level of communication skills. It can be
used as a self-assessment tool for the instructor to answer the question:
"During the experiential interview, did I model good communication skills?"
Of course, it also could be used to evaluate students' communication skills.

Providing Assistance

An instructor with good affective and communication skills is prepared
to provide assistance to the student to produce an affective behavior
change. In joint planning to achieve such a change, the faculty member
first demonstrates the affective skills of expressing empathy, demonstrating positive regard, and developing trust. The instructor then manifests
the communication skills of attending behavior, paraphrasing, reflecting
feeling, and summarizing content.

In initiating the effort, the instructor and student jointly define the
problem in an observable way. In overcoming behavioral problems, both
must agree on what the difficulty is. Both must believe a problem exists;
if they do, the potential behavior change will be worth the time and effort.

Once the problem has been defined, the desired behavior change must
be specified in an observable way. This will include answering the following questions:

1. *Who* is involved? Student? Faculty? Patients?
2. *What* is to be done? What is the desired behavioral change? Instructor
   and student must agree on a statement of purpose.
3. *Where* will the action take place? Home? School? Clinic? Hospital?

4. *How* can the behavior be performed? The instructor plans any new learning required and the tasks to be completed.
5. *When* are the actions to be performed? This should include a starting date and, if appropriate, a completion date.
6. *Why* is the student trying to modify a behavior? Will the change result in measurable benefits? Does the student understand the implications of the behavior change?

Once the commitments are made, the instructor must be able to provide support.

BEHAVIOR MODIFICATION INTERVIEW

The primary purpose of a behavior modification interview is to change a student's behavior. The techniques, theories, and principles of behavior modification are based upon operant conditioning. Operant conditioning is a type of learning that involves an increase in the probability of a response occurring as a function of reinforcement. The following is an excerpt from a behavior modification interview:

> *Instructor:* Your peers have told me that you are consistently rude to the patients.
> *Philip:* I just hate this clinical rotation. The nurses are not helpful and the patients are not motivated to get better.
> *Instructor:* Come now, you haven't given the rotation a chance. You've only been here three weeks.
> *Philip:* What do you know? You're not here all day!

So begins the behavior modification interview. The ultimate success of this and subsequent interviews may be very likely to determine Philip's success at his clinical rotation. This type of interview also requires a fairly unstructured format.

SUGGESTIONS FOR EFFECTIVE INTERVIEWING

The initial step is for the instructor to state the purpose of the interview. While the instructor may have one purpose, the student may have a different agenda. For example, during a conference regarding clinical performance, the student's primary purpose may be: "How can I get out of this clinical rotation?" The instructor's purpose may be: "How can I learn more about how Dan feels about his clinical performance to help make this a more satisfying experience for him, and for the hospital?"

The next step is to establish rapport with the student. When a student is greeted in a warm and friendly manner, is given a comfortable seat, and is extended the usual social courtesies, a good beginning is made. The instructor should sit facing the student so that eye contact is possible—if at all possible, not behind the desk. There should be no large physical barrier between the two.

As the third step, the instructor establishes a time limit for the interview. If the student feels pressure because of lack of time, the interview may be unsuccessful and should be rescheduled when time is not an inhibiting factor.

For the fourth step, the instructor should sharpen awareness of the barriers that inhibit a successful interview. Interrupting and prompting can inhibit the process and distort communication. For some reason the effective use of silence is difficult for people from Western cultures. However, instead of representing an absence of communication, silence can be a most effective form of communication. Knowing when to be silent is as important as knowing when to speak. The appropriate mix of listening and silence requires practice and patience.

There are no universal rules about how long silences should be. One effective technique is to allow the student to assume the responsibility for responding if that person initiated the silence. Students often need periods of silence to consider alternative courses of action, analyze feelings, and/ or evaluate a comment or decision.

Instructors should not be afraid of silence; used effectively, it can increase communication. Most persons in stressful situations (and interviews often are stressful) need time to prepare answers. An instructor may ask what a student thinks can be done to improve clinical performance. It may take a few moments to prepare a good answer. Those few minutes may seem like hours to the instructor. However, if the teacher interrupts the silence and presents a possible solution, the student has lost the opportunity to help cope with a personal problem. Silence also can encourage "active" listening.

The instructor, as the fifth step, practices the skillful use of questioning. This can promote thoughtfulness and encourage free expression. Carefully asked questions can encourage the flow of information. Questions can be used:

- To promote thoughtfulness: "How do you explain your behavior? What will be the probable outcome? What were you thinking about when it happened?"
- To express feelings: "How did you feel when the other person said no?"

- To redirect ideas: "You mentioned your father's influence on your behavior. Could you explain that further?"
- To aid exploration for more details: "You mentioned that the instructor is 'unfair.' What do you mean?"
- To clarify ambiguities or incomplete responses: "What did you mean when you said Jim spent a year 'licking his wounds?' "

When asking questions it is important to try to avoid using "why." That often implies faultfinding, impatience, and/or dissatisfaction. When the instructor asks, "Why did you fail to record the blood pressure?" the question suggests imposing blame rather than merely seeking information. A better course is to change "why" questions to "what" or "how." For example, "How do you think you could have increased the likelihood of patient compliance with your instructions?" is less apt to generate feelings of disapproval and blame.

Closed and open questions should be used appropriately. "Does the medication affect your ability to rest?" is a closed question, requesting either a "yes" or "no" answer. It unnecessarily restricts an answer. A more open question, "How does the medication affect your ability to rest or exercise?" encourages the patient to discuss the effects more fully. There are clear differences in the following closed/open questions:

- "Do you like to read? Tell me about your favorite leisure activities?"
- "Do you want your family to be told? How do you feel about discussing the abortion with your mother?"
- "Were you suprised about the outcome? What did you discover about yourself from the experience?"

The closed-ended questions focus the student's answer, the open ones leave room for the respondent to structure the answer. Both types of questions have their advantages and disadvantages. The skilled instructor knows how and when to use either or both.

The sixth step advises the instructor to choose the interview location with care. The environment should be relatively free from interruptions, especially the telephone. Nothing is more stifling to the flow of conversation than a telephone call, especially when the outcome is extremely important in the eyes of the student. Routine phone calls can be held until after the interview. Also, the location should be where the conversation cannot be overheard.

As the seventh step, the instructor must be prepared. A certain amount of preplanning precedes both structured and unstructured interviews. For example, carefully reviewing all of the information regarding the student in advance will enhance the probability that a correct decision will be made.

The instructor, as the eighth step, should obtain a basic knowledge in both communication theory and counseling techniques. This can increase the amount of information gleaned from an interview (Schulman, 1982). The affective skills of expressing empathy, demonstrating positive regard, and developing trust—in concert with the communication skills of attending behavior, paraphrasing, reflecting feeling, and summarizing content—will greatly enhance the likelihood of a successful interview.

The ninth recommendation is to avoid communicating a note of finality at the end of the interview. Regardless of the type of session, it should end with the message that there will be opportunities for other conferences if they seem desirable.

The instructor, at the tenth step, should remember that not all questions are requests for information. They often express an attitude or a feeling, or make a statement. For example:

"How do I look?"	This may be a search for acceptance.
"Do you think I'll ever be able to learn how to do this?"	This may be a search for encouragement.
"When will the grades be posted?"	This may be expressing worry about possible failure.

When questions in reality are expressions of an attitude, feeling, or concern but are answered as questions, the instructor has lost an opportunity to help the student.

The eleventh commandment to the instructor is to avoid offering direct advice. This gives students two options: they may follow the advice or not follow it. Some may ignore it because they may sense it is not appropriate to their circumstances, others may to maintain their independence. In contrast, students who follow advice may become dependent and blame the instructor if the results are not as expected. This blaming reduces the possibility that students will begin to make decisions for themselves and accept their consequences.

Finally, instructors must ground any hostile response to avoid the hostility/counterhostility cycle. There is an old but very valid saying: "Never answer an angry word with an angry word. It's the second one that makes the quarrel."

A hostile response is one that antagonizes or humiliates the student. Many educational programs are intense and create stress. Some students may respond to this stress by becoming irritated and projecting unreasonable demands on others, often becoming openly critical of the teaching staff. As a result, the teacher may react with counterhostility. For example, Sara might exclaim: "You don't care how many hours I spend in the intensive care unit. You just expect me to be there on time!" If the instructor does not respond defensively, the relationship will be free to develop in a positive way.

Interpreting Interview Data

Caution and common sense should be used when attempting to interpret interview data (Miller, 1962). The interview is only one piece of information and should not be used as the only criterion upon which to base a decision. All the following potential sources of bias should be considered:

- Interviewer bias: A cold, impersonal instructor will limit the amount of information exchanged but a warm, facilitative one will expand the information.
- Physical setting: An interview conducted in the instructor's office may bring responses different from one in the student's room.
- Student's anxiety level: This will affect performance during the interview.

There are a number of advantages in using the interview structure to deal with students' problems:

- Interviews are better than questionnaires for obtaining information that requires sequencing.
- Interviews can provide supplementary information to verify other material; this often is referred to as a "direct" method of determining attitude.
- Interviews permit flexibility by enabling the instructor to clarify questions, probe, and follow up in ways that are impossible in other forms.
- Interviews can be used effectively as the first step in the development of a questionnaire. Well-thought-out, probing interviews can provide the framework for a valid questionnaire (Henerson et al., 1978).
- Informal interviews may be a mechanism for diagnosing student problems.

Research on Interviews in General

The research on the general use of interviews may provide some insight into their effectiveness and their resultant validity and reliability. Anderson (1954) and Sydiaha (1962), when analyzing interviews through content analysis, report that interviewers control the length of the session more often than do interviewees; however, the latter have more control over the number of verbal exchanges.

Frank and Hackman (1975) find that the more similar the interviewee is to the interviewer, the more likely it is that a favorable session will be recorded. The factors included sex; socioeconomic level; type of schooling; urban or rural background; intellectual pursuits; interest in athletics, art, and hobbies; and organizational memberships.

Huse (1962) says that the ability to predict job success based on the interview is as high as the ability to predict job success using psychometric tests.

Mann (1977) shows only a weak positive relationship between interview performance and field work performance for occupation therapy students. In contrast, many of the studies concerning interviewer reliability do not give correlation coefficients. However, Anderson (1954), Mann (1977), Prien (1962), and Shaw (1952) report reliability coefficients ranging from 0.52 through 0.80.

While there is general agreement that interviews are not the best predictors of success, they can be used effectively to provide input into such areas as clinical evaluation and general attitudes toward the clinical environment. Mann (1977) regards the interview as extremely useful for measuring interpersonal skills and career motivation.

ADAPTING TRADITIONAL EVALUATION METHODS*

Traditional evaluation methods can be used to assess affective objectives. Both objective and essay-type test items can be written. Objective test items can be divided into two kinds: (1) "supply-type" objective items that require students to supply short answers and to complete test items, and (2) "selection-type" objective items that require students to choose a response (agree/disagree and multiple choice items). Essay-type items also have a legitimate place in evaluation.

Developing evaluation methods for affective objectives identifies the affective domain as an indispensable and legitimate area of learning. This section analyzes supply-type, selection-type, and essay objective items, including guidelines for writing test items and sample items.

---

*Adapted from King, E.C. Constructing classroom achievement tests. *Nurse Educator,* 1978, *3*, 30–36. Copyright © 1978 with permission of *Nurse Educator.*

SUPPLY-TYPE TEST ITEMS

The supply-type test item has two major advantages: it minimizes the likelihood of correct guessing and is relatively easy to construct. However, it has major weaknesses. It often is difficult to score because of the variety of correct and partially correct answers.

In writing supply-type items, instructors should be careful to avoid using statements verbatim from textbooks and other sources. They also should avoid eliminating so many words that clairvoyance is needed to answer the statement. Blanks should be placed near the end of the statement, not at the beginning.

Objective

(For all examples in this final section of the chapter, the learners in the Objective are the nursing students, so only the behavior at issue is stated.)

Apply the communication skills of paraphrasing and reflection of feeling.

> *Test Item*
> "I've tried and tried to make friends since coming here but I still do not feel that anybody cares."
> Paraphrase the above response:
>
> _____
>
> _____ .
>
> Formulate your response to the expression of feeling:
> "You feel _____ .

Alternative Response Items

The most common form of the alternate response is the agree/disagree or accept/not accept item. It can be used to ascertain beliefs and attitudes characteristic of the awareness and responding level of the affective domain. To increase the depth and breadth of the responding level, students also can be asked to further explain a rationale or define a choice.

In writing alternative response test items, instructors should avoid using "specific determiners" such as "only," "all," "never," "generally," "often," and "sometimes." It also is important to keep items relatively short and restricted to one central idea. Carefully written directions are essential.

> *Directions:*
> For each of the following circle "A" if you agree with the statement and "D" if you don't agree.

1. The quality of nursing care for the attempted suicide patient is different from that required for the terminally ill cancer patient.   A   D
2. Patients should be allowed to die without excessive intervention methods to support life if this is their desire.   A   D

Special Alternative Response Items

The alternative response item can be expanded by relating it to some given material (for example, a chart or patient case study). This kind of item allows the instructor to ascertain the class's commonly held belief and attitudes more effectively (Exhibit 4-18).

Exhibit 4-18 Alternate Response Type Item*

Maria is a 6-year-old child with chronic renal failure. She has been suffering from progressive, inexorable nephron destruction for almost a year. At present she is being maintained on antibiotics and fluid restrictions, along with constraints in phosphorus, electrolytes, and nitrogen in her diet. She needs hemodialysis three times a week even with the strict dietary restrictions. Transplantation is being considered as a last resort to allow Maria to live a normal life. Consents have been obtained and the family is awaiting a donor.

Keith is an 8-year-old boy brought to the emergency room with severe head trauma following a car accident. His condition is extremely critical and he is not expected to live through the night. The nephrologist speaks with the family regarding possible donation of Keith's kidneys in the event he should die. He tells Keith's family about the many children waiting for a kidney so they can live normal lives. The doctor is unaware that Keith's mother is a nurse and his father a hematologist. The parents refuse to donate Keith's kidneys. They want all extraordinary measures to be taken to try to save Keith's life, regardless of the possible brain damage. The mother declares that she does not believe doctors wait for a patient to die before they take organs. She believes patients are even left to die so that others might live; and anyway, what right does the doctor have to make a decision that her son isn't worth saving?

Directions:
Circle A if you agree with the statement and D if you disagree.
1. Keith's parents do not trust physicians.   A   D
2. Maria should have a kidney transplant.   A   D
3. I would donate Keith's kidneys if he died if I were his parents.   A   D
4. Letting Keith die is more consistent with respect and compassion than using heroic measures when severe brain damage is obvious.   A   D
5. All extraordinary measures should be taken to save Keith's life, regardless of the brain damage.   A   D

*The author acknowledges that Joanna F. Hofmann, R.N., gave her permission to use this true case study. Patient names have been changed to protect their confidentiality.

It should be noted carefully that while the alternate response item is useful in determining attitudes, misconceptions, and beliefs, these affective items should not be translated into grades. If the instructor asks the students to explain or defend their choice(s) in writing, the written paragraph may be graded for such things as spelling, punctuation, sentence construction, concepts of good grammar, and flow of ideas. However, the content of the response should not be graded.

Multiple-Choice Test Items

The multiple-choice test item is one in which an incomplete statement is presented and a number of possible responses or options are given. The question or incomplete statement introducing the item is called the stem. An incorrect answer is called a distractor or a foil. Exhibit 4-19 illustrates the parts of a multiple-choice question.

The outstanding feature of this item is its versatility. Its primary limitation is that it often is time consuming and difficult to build. However, its advantages far outweigh these limitations. Since writing good multiple-choice items takes much time and thought, many nursing instructors do not allow their exams to be freely distributed; students are allowed to review them in the teacher's office. Consequently, the instructor does not have to completely rewrite them each semester.

GUIDELINES FOR MULTIPLE-CHOICE ITEMS

In writing multiple-choice examinations, the instructor first should select foils that are plausible to those who do not know the content demanded

---

Exhibit 4-19 Parts of a Multiple-Choice Question

Objective: Willingness of nurse to allocate decision making to patient(s).
Test Item:
Susan A. has been admitted following a car accident. She appears very depressed but is not seriously injured. Her brother arrives and asks your permission to take Susan to see her mother, who also is in the hospital and is not expected to recover. Susan seems anxious to see her mother. Who should decide whether Susan visits her mother?

1. Susan, the patient (Correct Answer)
2. You, the nurse (Foil/Distractor)
3. The brother (Foil/Distractor)
4. The mother (Foil/Distractor)
5. The physician (Foil/Distractor)

by the item. The number of available choices should be varied from at least three to not more than five. The length of the option must not be related to the tendency to be correct.

As much information as possible should be placed in the stem. All choices (correct answer and foils) must be grammatically consistent with the stem. Each item must be independent of the others so students cannot deduce subsequent answers on the basis of earlier questions.

There are three basic varieties of multiple-choice items—the negative, the multiple response, and the combined response.

Negative

There are many times when the use of negative wording is basic to the measurement of learning. Knowing what should not be said or done is so important it often requires negative emphasis. Many nursing procedures and interactions place some emphasis on practices to be avoided. However, since negative expressions in the stem can present difficult reading problems to students, the negative wording should be emphasized by underlining or the use of CAPITAL letters. It should be kept in mind that the primary objective of testing is to measure learning outcomes, not to trick students. For example:

Test Item
What is a common response of nurses working with incurably ill patients that should NOT be permitted:

1. psychological abandonment
2. aggressive treatment
3. passive euthanasia.

Multiple Response

In a multiple-response question, there may be as few as one or as many as five correct answers. To avoid possible confusion, the instructor must write clear, concise directions if multiple-response items are used (Exhibit 4-20).

Combined Response

The combined-response multiple-choice (Exhibit 4-21) item is effective in measuring students' ability to analyze, evaluate, and solve problems. It often is more difficult to answer and more discriminating than the typical form of multiple-choice items (Hughes & Trimble, 1965).

Exhibit 4-20 A Multiple-Response Item

Directions:
One or more than one response may be correct. Please circle ALL correct responses.
Objective: Apply the communication skill of reflection of feeling.
Test Item:
Which of the following response(s) appropriately reflects the feelings of Ruth, a young nursing student, when she says, "I really want to help Mr. Vittetoe, my first cardiac patient, but as soon as I get one problem sorted out and a patient care plan proposed he 'yes, buts' and has several reasons why he cannot do what we worked out." [Numbers of correct answers below are italicized.]

1. "Some people are no damn good."
2. "You feel frustrated because you have carefully explored the alternatives with Mr. Vittetoe and yet he will not accept any responsibility for his problem."
3. "You feel angry that nothing you propose seems to satisfy Mr. Vittetoe."
4. "You just lay down the law to him. He does it your way or else."
5. "Mr. Vittetoe is a pain. Give him your best advice and forget about him."

ESSAY TEST ITEMS

The most significant features of the essay test item are the freedom of expression and creativity allowed students and the emphasis on depth and breadth of knowledge. It also requires students to organize knowledge into a coherent whole. However, the essay test item has many major limitations: (1) representative sampling of course content is limited, (2)

Exhibit 4-21 A Combined Response Item

Objective: Support a quadriplegic individual in expressing grief.
Test Item
Which of the following response(s) supports the feeling of grief in a patient who says: "I don't know. Nothing seems to be going well for me. Who can love a quad?" [Correct answer numbers are in italic.]

1. Sounds like you're feeling frustrated and are very angry.
2. You should be happy that you survived the car accident, two others died.
3. You feel disappointed because things are not progressing as you had hoped.
4. You should explore your potential with our rehabilitation counselor.
5. You're afraid that your accident is going to change how people feel about you.

- 2 and 4
- 1 and 3
- *1, 3, and 5*
- None of the above.

---

good items can be difficult to write, (3) scoring often is difficult, unreliable, and time consuming, and may require a content expert. Even with these limitations, the essay test item can be an effective evaluation tool for the affective taxonomy (King, 1979).

It should be remembered that if an opinion or philosophical stand is asked for, the grading should cover the students' ability to analyze, synthesize, and evaluate data, not the content of the item. Exhibit 4-22 illustrates sample evaluation criteria for scoring an essay item (King, 1979).

GUIDELINES FOR WRITING ESSAY TEST ITEMS

There are, as with the other types, some guidelines for writing essay test items (King, 1979) (Exhibits 4-23, 4-24, and 4-25). The instructor should write both the directions and the items in clear, precise language. All students should be required to answer the same item. Adequate time

---

Exhibit 4-22 Criteria for Evaluating Essay Questions

1. *Writing Mechanics* (25 points)
   The following will be used to evaluate writing mechanics:

   - Proper use of capitalization
   - Proper use of punctuation
   - Use of complete sentences
   - Appropriate use of simple, complex, and compound sentences
   - Relationship among sentences within paragraphs
   - Relationship among paragraphs (adequate transitions between paragraphs)
   - Appropriate sequence of paragraphs
   - Unity and smoothness
   - Organization of paper with appropriate subheadings, footnotes, bibliography, etc.; proper use of style (i.e., *The Chicago Manual of Style* (13th ed., 1982) or other accepted style format).

2. *Content* (75 points)

   - Clear statement of objective(s), problems, and boundaries of the selected topic
   - Evidence of careful literature review and search
   - Documentation of ideas
   - Identification of personal opinions, when expressed
   - Consideration of depth and breadth of analysis
   - Logical summary and conclusions following from the body of the paper.

Source: Adapted from *Classroom Evaluation Strategies* by Elizabeth C. King, published by The C.V. Mosby Company, St. Louis. Copyright © 1979, by permission of The C.V. Mosby Company.

Exhibit 4-23 Example of an Essay Test Item*

Objective:
Develop an awareness that an individual's value system influences behavior and decisions.
Test Item

Mr. and Mrs. Phillips visited the doctor and requested amniocentesis. Their first child, a daughter, had been born with isolated cleft lip and palate. The defect was repaired surgically and there was minimal scarring. They were concerned about problems with their second child. Mrs. Phillips, age 28, was now three months pregnant.

The doctor did a careful review of family history and explained to the parents that hereditary defects can appear even with no known familial pattern. He listened to the parents and allowed them to verbalize the sadness and guilt they experienced when their daughter was born. The doctor reinforced what others had told them: that they were not guilty of some "sin" because they had a deformed child, even though the deformity was mild and was well corrected. The doctor scheduled amniocentesis for the following week.

After the procedure, the parents visited the doctor's office again to hear the results. The doctor happily told them their expected child was normal in every way and they could look forward to a healthy baby girl in five months.

When the parents went home, they discussed the possibility of an abortion. They felt that could afford to raise only two children at the most, and really wanted a boy.

Mrs. Phillips had an abortion three days later.*

1. Based on the decision of Mr. and Mrs. Phillips, what inferences can be made regarding their personal value system?
2. If you were Mrs. Phillips, what would you have done? Why?

*The author acknowledges that Joanna F. Hofmann, R.N., gave her permission to use this true case. Patient names have been changed to protect their confidentiality.

should be provided for them to respond to the item. If necessary because of lack of time, the students could be allowed to answer as an out-of-class assignment. If the response is to be graded, the student should be informed as to the basis for the evaluation.

SCORING ESSAY TEST ITEMS

The essay test item emphasizes the holistic approach because it can integrate both the affective and the cognitive domains, requiring the student to function at a high cognitive level. This high-level mental process can be focused on a specified set of learning objectives. The most recurrent criticism of the essay test item, as noted earlier, is its scoring unreliability.

Exhibit 4-24 Another Type of Essay Test Item

Objective:
Protect the confidentiality of patient records.
Directions:
Select the response (1, 2, or 3) that you believe is the most correct and discuss the principle that supports your conclusion. If you believe the "best" response is inadequate, formulate a better one. Discuss the rationale for your improved response and the principle that supports that conclusion. For each of the options you have *not* chosen, discuss: (1) the principle on which you rejected it and (2) the possible consequence(s) if the response were given.
Test Item

It is five minutes from quitting time, the phone rings, and you answer it. "This is Mr. Hovey, from the Legal Aid Society," the caller says. "Do you have the barbiturate test results on Ms. Dorothy R. today?"

You check the records and find the test results are recorded. After telling Mr. Hovey the test is complete, he says he is preparing Ms. R.'s defense for the custody trial for her two preschool children. He needs the results as soon as possible and will accept responsibility for their being given over the telephone.

You say:
1. "The test is finished but I'm not sure the results have been verified."
2. "I'll have Mrs. R.'s physician return your call."
3. "The result is 80 grams/ml."

Its practical value may be limited by the instructor's inability to score the item reliably. For example, an instructor may rate a response as a B + but after reading the response a second time may rate the response as a C +. Furthermore, two different instructors may rate the response differently. However a mixture of essay and objective test items improves reliability and enhances content validity.

The following procedure for rating or scoring essay responses is suggested (King, 1979). The instructor should:

1. Construct a sample response. The preparation of a model answer is difficult but not impossible. After a model has been prepared, it should be checked against a sample of student responses. If it is found that the students' replies consistently differ from the model answer, then it should be revised. Some instructors object to this procedure on the ground that it lowers academic standards. However, as Thorndike and Hagen (1969) point out, the discrepancy between responses may result from poor directions, poorly designed test item(s), or expectations that are unrealistic in light of students' previous learning or the limits of testing time.

Exhibit 4-25 Essay Question on Kohlberg's Theory*

Objective:
Apply Kohlberg's theory of cognitive moral development to a controversial issue.
Background:
Mrs. Smith has just returned from the operating room after a radical hysterectomy for cancer of the cervix. During surgery doctors noted extensive metastasis to the liver, spleen, and intestines. A colon resection and an illeostomy were performed. Mrs. Smith was scheduled to undergo extensive radiation and chemotherapy even though her prognosis was poor, with a life expectancy of six to eight months.

Mr. Smith asked why the illeostomy was performed if his wife only had a few months to live anyway. The surgeon explained that the intestinal tumors were large and widespread and would cause excessive pain and nausea and even shorten the limited life expectancy by causing a total intestinal obstruction.

Mr. Smith did not want his wife to know her prognosis. He said she was the type who would give up if she felt there was no hope.

A few days after the surgery, Mrs. Smith asked the nurse if her illeostomy would be permanent. The nurse said she didn't know but she would find out. She never returned with the answer. The night nurse, not knowing the family's request, honestly answered Mrs. Smith's questions, although she did not tell her the prognosis.

The next day Mr. Smith became outraged when he discovered the night nurse had told Mrs. Smith her illeostomy was permanent.

Test Item:
Should the night nurse have answered Mrs. Smith's question? According to Kohlberg, various responses to the question would be given at various levels of cognitive moral development. (1) Describe each level and stage of Kohlberg's moral development theory and (2) give an example of a possible response to the question at each level.

*The author acknowledges that Joanna F. Hofmann, R.N., gave her permission to use this true case. Patient names have been changed to protect their confidentiality.

2. State clearly the criteria for evaluating the answer.
3. Read responses one at a time, sorting them into piles that represent the letter grades expected to be assigned. During the first reading, answers that do not clearly fall into any grade category should be identified with a question mark and placed in the apparently closest pile.
4. Reread each response, giving special attention to the papers carrying a question mark.
5. Repeat Steps 3 and 4 for each essay item.
6. Be especially careful, if the item deals with a controversial issue, to evaluate it in terms of the "presentation of evidence" for the position chosen rather than the choice itself.

7. Shuffle the papers after scoring each response because instructors may find the grading of a paper may be influenced by the quality of the previous response. For example, Jennifer writes superior answers to each essay question while Jim's responses are average. If the instructor reads Jim's adequate responses after Jennifer's, Jim's all may appear below average. To prevent Jim's overall grade from being lowered almost automatically by this potential instructor bias, the papers should be shuffled to vary the scoring sequence.
8. Tally the letter grades for each essay item and assign an overall letter grade.

As King (1979) states:

> While the rating method is recommended for grading essay items, it is not very reliable. When reading essay responses, instructors should concentrate on correcting errors and writing comments. Carefully scored essay items maximize student motivation and learning. It is far better to carefully prepare and score one item then to cursorily score five. Carefully considered written comments can be another excellent mechanism for increasing student motivation. Thorough feedback is more effective than most instructors realize. It is like a private conversation between instructor and student and is highly valued by students.

This discussion has been designed to assist nursing instructors in adapting traditional evaluation methods to the assessment of affective objectives. Evaluation items must mirror the instructor's objectives. There must be congruence between the behavioral objective and the evaluation procedure. Since the affective domain is a significant component in the practice of nursing, it also should be present in the development of objectives and the evaluation procedures.

REFERENCES

Abrams, R.G., & Kelly, M.L. Student self-evaluation in a pediatric-operative technique course. *Journal of Dental Education,* 1974, *38*(7), 385–391.

Amatora, M. Validity in self-evaluation. *Educational and Psychological Measurement,* 1956, *16,* 119–126.

Anderson, R.C. The guided interview as an evaluative instrument. *The Journal of Educational Research,* Nov. 1954, *48,* 203–209.

Berdie, R.F. Self-claimed and test knowledge. *Educational and Psychological Measurement* 1971, *31,* 629–636.

Bernstein, L.B.; Bernstein, R.S.; & Dana, R.H. *Interviewing: A guide for health professionals* (2nd ed.). New York: Appleton-Century-Crofts, Inc., 1974.

Carkhuff, R.R. *Helping and human relations: A primer for lay and professional helpers* (Vols. 1 and 2). New York: Holt, Rinehart & Winston, Inc., 1969.

Dohner, C.W. Rating scales in clinical evaluation. In D.M. Irby & M.K. Morgan (Eds.), *Clinical evaluation: Alternatives for health-related educators.* Gainesville, Fla.: University of Florida, Center for Allied Health Personnel, 1974.

Ebel, R.C. The relation of scale finesse to grade accuracy. *Journal of Educational Measurement,* Winter 1969, *6,* 217–221.

Ekman, P., & Friesen, W. Nonverbal leakage and clues to perception. *Psychiatry,* 1969, *32,* 88–106.

Frank, L., & Hackman, J.R. Effects of interviewer-interviewee similarity on interviewer objectivity in college admissions interviews. *Journal of Applied Psychology,* 1975, *60*(3), 356.

Gaier, E.L. Student self-estimates of final course grades. *The Journal of Genetic Psychology,* 1966, *98,* 63–67.

Geissler, P.R. Student self-assessment in dental technology. *Journal of Dental Education,* September 1973, *37*(9), 19–21.

Gilmore, J.B. Learning and student self-evaluation. *Journal of College Science Teaching,* October 1973, *3*(1), 54–57.

Gordon, M.J. Assessment of student affect: A clinical approach. In M.K. Morgan & D.M. Irby (Eds.), *Evaluating clinical competence in the health professions.* St. Louis: The C.V. Mosby Company, 1978.

Grussing, P.G.; Silzer, R.F.; & Cyrs, T.E., Jr. Development of behaviorally anchored rating scales for pharmacy practice. *American Journal of Pharmaceutical Education,* May 1979, *43*(2), 115–120.

Guilford, J.P. *Psychometric methods* (2nd ed.). New York: McGraw-Hill Book Company, 1954.

Hanson, P.G. What to look for in groups. In J.W. Pfeiffer & J.E. Jones (Eds.), *The 1972 annual handbook for group facilitators.* San Diego: University Associates, Inc., 1972.

Henerson, M.E.; Morris, L.L.; & Fitz-Gibbon, C.T. *How to measure attitudes.* Beverly Hills, Calif.: Sage Publications, Inc., 1978.

Hovland, C.I., & Sherif, M. Judgmental phenomena and scales of attitude measurement: Item displacement in Thurstone scales. *Journal of Abnormal and Social Psychology,* 1952, *47,* 822–832.

Hughes, H., & Trimble, W. The use of complex alternatives in multiple-choice items. *Educational and Psychological Measurement,* 1965, *25,* 117–126.

Huse, E. Assessments of higher level personnel: IV, The validity of assessment techniques based on systematically varied information. *Personnel Psychology* 1962, *15,* 195–205.

Irby, D.M., & Dohner, C.W. Student clinical performance. In C.W. Ford & M.K. Morgan (Eds.), *Teaching in the health professions.* St. Louis: The C.V. Mosby Company, 1976.

Kendon, A. Some relationships between body motion and speech: An analysis of an example. In A. Siegman & B. Pope (Eds.), *Studies in dyadic communication.* London: Pergamon Co., 1972.

King, E.C. Constructing classroom achievement tests. *Nurse Educator,* September-October 1978, *3,* 30–36.

King, E.C. *Classroom evaluation strategies.* St. Louis: The C.V. Mosby Company, 1979.

Lemon, N. *Attitudes and their measurement.* New York: John Wiley & Sons, Inc., 1973.

Likert, R. A technique for measurement of attitudes. *Archives of Psychology,* 1932, *140.*

Lindeman, R. *Educational measurement.* Glenview, Ill.: Scott, Foresman & Company, 1967.

Mager, R.F. *Preparing instructional objectives.* Palo Alto, Calif.: Pacific Book Publishers, 1968.

Mann, W.C. *Reliability of evaluative interviews for admission into health professional training.* Unpublished doctoral dissertation, State University of New York at Buffalo, 1977.

Marriner, A. Student self-evaluation and the contracted grade. *Nursing Forum,* Spring 1974, *13.*

Mehrabian, A. *Nonverbal communication.* Chicago: Atherton Co., 1972.

Miller, G.E. (Ed.). *Teaching and learning in medical schools.* Cambridge, Mass.: Harvard University Press, 1962.

Osgood, C.E. Cross cultural comparability in attitude research via multilingual semantic differentials. In Steiner, I. & Fishbein, M. (eds.), *Current studies in social psychology.* New York: Holt, Rinehart and Winston, 1965.

Osgood, C.E.; Suci, G.J.; & Tannenbaum, P.H. *The measurement of meaning.* Urbana, Ill.: The University of Illinois Press, 1957.

Prien, E.P. Assessment of higher-level personnel: V, An analysis of interviewers' prediction of job performance. *Personnel Psychology,* 1962, *15,* 319–334.

Risser, N.L. Risser patient satisfaction scale. In M.J. Ward & C. Lindeman (Eds.), *Instruments for measuring nursing practice and other health care variables* (Vol. 2). Hyattsville, Md.: U.S. Department of Health, Education, and Welfare, Public Health Service, Health Resources Administration, ed. 3, n.d.

Schulman, E.D. *Intervention in human services.* St. Louis: The C.V. Mosby Company, 1982.

Sergiovanni, T.J. *Handbook for effective department leadership: Concepts and practices in today's secondary schools.* Boston: Allyn & Bacon, Inc., 1977.

Shaw, J. The function of the interview in determining fitness for teacher training. *Journal of Educational Research,* 1952, *45,* 667–681.

Skinner, B.F. *Contingencies of reinforcement.* New York: Appleton-Century-Crofts, Inc., 1969.

Sydiaha, D. Bales interaction process analysis of personnel selection interviews. *Journal of Applied Psychology,* 1962, *44,* 344–349.

Thorndike, R.L., & Hagen, E. *Measurement and evaluation in psychology and education* (3rd ed.). New York: John Wiley & Sons, Inc., 1969.

Thurstone, L.L. Rank order as a psychophysical method. *Journal of Experimental Psychology,* 1931, *14,* 187–201.

Thurstone, L.L. *The measurement of values* (4th Impression). Chicago: The University of Chicago Press, 1967.

Truax, C.B., & Carkhuff, R.R. *Toward effective counseling and psychotherapy.* Chicago: Aldine Publishing Co., Inc., 1967.

Warr, P.B., & Knapper, C. *The perception of people and events.* New York: John Wiley & Sons, Inc., 1968.

Wells, W.D., & Smith, G. Four semantic scales compared. *Journal of Applied Psychology,* 1960, *44,* 393–397.

Wittich, W.A., & Schuller, C.F. *Instructional technology: Its nature and use* (5th ed.). New York: Harper and Row, Publishers, Inc., 1973.

Wrightstone, W.J.; Justman, J.; & Robbins, I. *Evaluation in modern education.* New York: The American Book Company, 1956.

Appendix 4-A

Sample Likert-Type Scale

RISSER PATIENT SATISFACTION SCALE

This questionnaire is designed to find out what kinds of things patients like or don't like about the nursing care they receive in their doctors' offices. Your ideas, along with those of other patients, will be used to try to improve the care you are now receiving here.

This questionnaire contains a number of statements, each of which says something different about nurses. For each statement, decide how much you agree or disagree with the view expressed. Think about the care you are now receiving here as you respond to each statement. In a column next to the statements you will find five words to use to describe your opinion. Circle the number under the word which comes closest to your own opinion. There are no right or wrong answers. People differ in their views. Your response is a matter of your personal opinion.

People here at _____ know that I am asking for your help. But no one here will see the way you answer the questionnaire. The information you give me will be completely confidential.

If, for any reason, you do not feel you are able to complete this questionnaire, please feel free to hand it back to me unfinished.

Thank you very much for your time and your help. Below is an example which may help you in completing the questionnaire.

Source: Reprinted from *Instruments for Measuring Nursing Practice and Other Health Care Variables,* Vol. 2, by Nancy Risser (M.J. Ward and C. Lindeman, Eds.), U.S. Department of Health, Education, and Welfare, n.d., with permission of the author.

	Strongly Agree	Agree	Neutral	Disagree	Strongly Disagree
A. The nurse thinks I understand more than I really do.	①	2	3	4	5
B. Nurses are put in the position of needing to know more than they possibly could.	1	2	③	4	5

The answer to question A indicates that you are quite certain that the nurse thinks you understand more than you really do. The answer to question B, "neutral," indicates you can't quite decide whether to agree or to disagree with this statement.

Circle the number under the word which comes closest to your own opinion. PLEASE BE SURE TO MARK EVERY STATEMENT.

	Strongly Agree	Agree	Neutral	Disagree	Strongly Disagree
1. The nurse is skillful in assisting the doctor with procedures.	1	2	3	4	5
2. The nurse is understanding in listening to a patient's problems.	1	2	3	4	5
3. The nurse really knows what she is talking about.	1	2	3	4	5
4. The nurse doesn't always tell me what effects to expect from my drugs like she could.	1	2	3	4	5

	Strongly Agree	Agree	Neutral	Disagree	Strongly Disagree
5. The nurse explains things in simple language.	1	2	3	4	5
6. It is always easy to understand what the nurse is talking about.	1	2	3	4	5
7. The nurse should be more attentive than she is.	1	2	3	4	5
8. The nurse is just not patient enough.	1	2	3	4	5
9. The nurse is not precise in doing her work.	1	2	3	4	5
10. When I need to talk to someone, I can go to the nurse with my problems.	1	2	3	4	5
11. The nurse is too busy at the desk to spend time talking with me.	1	2	3	4	5
12. The nurse makes it a point to show me how to carry out the doctor's orders.	1	2	3	4	5
13. The nurse is too slow to do things for me.	1	2	3	4	5
14. The nurse is pleasant to be around.	1	2	3	4	5
15. The nurse forgets to make sure that I know how and when to take my medicine.	1	2	3	4	5
16. The nurse is often too disorganized to appear calm.	1	2	3	4	5

	Strongly Agree	Agree	Neutral	Disagree	Strongly Disagree
17. Too often the nurse thinks you can't understand the medical explanation of your illness, so she just doesn't bother to explain.	1	2	3	4	5
18. The nurse always gives complete enough explanations of why tests are ordered.	1	2	3	4	5
19. I'm tired of the nurse talking down to me.	1	2	3	4	5
20. The nurse is a person who can understand how I feel.	1	2	3	4	5
21. The nurse gives directions too fast.	1	2	3	4	5
22. The nurse gives good advice over the telephone.	1	2	3	4	5
23. The nurse should be more friendly than she is.	1	2	3	4	5
24. I wish the nurse would tell me about the results of my tests more than she does.	1	2	3	4	5
25. The nurse asks a lot of questions, but once she finds the answers, she doesn't seem to do anything.	1	2	3	4	5
26. The nurse gives directions at just the right speed.	1	2	3	4	5

	Strongly Agree	Agree	Neutral	Disagree	Strongly Disagree
27. A person feels free to ask the nurse questions.	1	2	3	4	5
28. Just talking to the nurse makes me feel better.	1	2	3	4	5

Appendix 4-B

Checklist for New Administrators

Directions:

Individuals new to a leadership role often are concerned with common problems. Check "Yes" or "No" on the common problems listed below. Check "N.A." when "Yes" or "No" would be inappropriate or not applicable. If you check "Yes" for any of the problems, discuss these with a good friend in a leadership position.

	Does this problem affect you?			
Common Problems	*Yes*	*No*	*N.A.*	*Comment*
1. You may feel uneasy. Many factors contribute to a general feeling of uneasiness in a leadership position. Although others have expressed confidence in you, you may have some self-doubt about your ability to do the job.	_____	_____	_____	_____
2. Your job description is generally vague; the higher up in the organization you go, the less specific your job description. More time is spent making				

Source: Adapted from *Handbook for Effective Department Leadership: Concepts and Practices in Today's Secondary Schools* by Thomas J. Sergiovanni, published by Allyn & Bacon, Inc., Boston. Copyright © 1977, by permission of Allyn & Bacon, Inc.

	Does this problem affect you?			
Common Problems	*Yes*	*No*	*N.A.*	*Comment*

decisions than performing specific job-related tasks. Innovation and initiative are expected. Job security may not be available. The workday often extends into the evening. Your performance is more visible to others. Can you deal with this ambiguity? ____ ____ ____ _____

3. You may have difficulty with confidential information. As a new leader you have access to a much wider information network. However, much of this information is confidential. Do you ever feel frustrated because you are unable to share this information? ____ ____ ____ _____

4. You are not readily accepted as one of the group. Some of your decisions may cause hard feelings among the staff. This will separate you somewhat. Even if you have high affiliation needs, this may not be possible. Are you ready to accept the consequences of your "unpopular" decisions? ____ ____ ____ _____

5. You are concerned about filling another's shoes. People will have expectations about your performance. There may be some rather cool interpersonal reactions until they are secure with your style. Are you willing to be patient? ____ ____ ____ _____

	Does this problem affect you?			
Common Problems	Yes	No	N.A.	Comment
6. The higher you go, the less specialized your job tasks. Health care providers often are specialists. As they move into supervisory positions their role becomes more that of a generalist. They will need to understand such areas as budget planning, management, and the relationship between the department and the entire institution. Can you change your role from a specialist to a generalist?	_____	_____	_____	_____
7. You may experience some role conflict. You cannot always please everyone. Yet most hospital organizational structures identify the supervisor as part health care professional, part administrator. The staff will expect you to implement its policy decisions. At times these two expectations may be in conflict. Can you cope with this role conflict?	_____	_____	_____	_____

Appendix 4-C

Checklist for Effective Group Functioning

When building an effective group, the concern is not only with identifying goals and objectives but also with the interpersonal side of group functioning. For groups to be effective, the members should share common objectives. This also helps contribute to high task effectiveness. The effective group also is a psychological entity: if its members enjoy interacting with each other, identify with the group, and find membership satisfying, this psychological component also will contribute to group effectiveness (Sergiovanni, 1977).

To build and maintain high effectiveness, attention to such group traits as morale, atmosphere, participation, styles of influence, leadership, conflict, and cooperation is important. Increasing sensitivity to these traits can help individuals (administrators, instructors) identify potential problems and deal with them more effectively.

WHAT TO LOOK FOR IN GROUP BEHAVIOR*

Maintenance Functions

These functions are crucial to the morale of the group. They maintain good and harmonious working relationships and help the group deal with the discussion of complex issues. For example, when decisions are being made on a controversial issue, these maintenance functions help the group "solve" the problem without seriously destroying its morale and effec-

---

*Adapted from Pfeiffer, J.W., & Jones, J.E. (Eds). *The 1972 Annual Handbook for Group Facilitators* (Contributed by P.G. Hanson, V.A. Hospital, Texas). San Diego: University Associates, © 1972. Used by permission.

tiveness. Maintenance functions ensure effective teamwork within the group.

The maintenance functions observation form shown in Exhibit 4C-1 is a checklist that helps the observer identify which group members help others (1) get into the conversion (gatekeepers), (2) summarize group feeling, and (3) mediate conflict. The definitions of the traits to be observed follow (the numbers refer to the functions as listed in Exhibit 4C-1):

Exhibit 4C-1 Maintenance Functions Observation Checklist

Directions:
1. Observer should be familiar with the maintenance functions as defined in the [accompanying] "Definition of Terms Used on Maintenance Function Observation Checklist."
2. Each group member's name should be recorded in space definitions provided on the checklist.
3. Each time a member performs a "Maintenance Function," a slash or checkmark should be placed in the appropriate box.

Maintenance Function	Group Members' Names				
	Edmund	Pauline	Larry	Eileen	Mary
1. Harmonizing		I	IIII	I	IIII
2. Gatekeeping				I	II
3. Consensus Testing					II
4. Encouraging		IIII IIII			II
5. Compromising		IIII IIII			II
6. Following		IIII IIII			
7. Expressing Group Feeling				IIII IIII IIII	IIII
8. Mediating					IIII
9. Relieving Tension		IIII IIII IIII	III	I	IIII
10. Other					

Source: Adapted from J.W. Pfeiffer and J.E. Jones (eds.), *The 1972 Annual Handbook for Group Facilitators.* Contributed by Philip G. Hanson, V.A. Hospital, Houston, Tex. San Diego, Calif.: University Associates, 1972. Used with permission.

1. **Harmonizing:** attempting to reconcile disagreements, reducing differences or getting people to explore them.
2. **Gatekeeping:** helping to keep communication channels open, facilitating the participation of others, suggesting procedures that permit sharing remarks.
3. **Consensus Testing:** asking to see whether group is nearing a decision, sending up trial balloon to test a possible conclusion.
4. **Encouraging:** being friendly, warm, and responsive to others; indicating by facial expression or remark the acceptance of others' contributions.
5. **Compromising:** offering a compromise that yields status, admitting error, making modifications in the interest of group cohesion or growth, when own idea or status is involved in a conflict.
6. **Following:** going along with decisions of the group, accepting ideas of others thoughtfully, serving as audience during group discussion.
7. **Expressing Group Feeling:** summarizing what group feeling is sensed to be, describing reactions of the group to ideas or solutions.
8. **Mediating:** conciliating differences in points of view, making compromise solutions.
9. **Relieving Tension:** draining off negative feelings by jesting or pouring oil on troubled waters, putting a tense situation in wider context.

From the observations checked in Exhibit 4C-1 it may be concluded that:

1. Edmund did not participate in any group maintenance functions.
2. Pauline was active in encouraging (i.e., being friendly, warm, and responsive to others), compromising (i.e., when her ideas were involved in a conflict she was willing to compromise, admit error, or modify the ideas in the interest of group cohesion and growth) and following (thoughtfully accepting the ideas of others).
3. Larry was active in harmonizing (i.e., attempting to reconcile disagreements) and in relieving tension (i.e., draining off negative feelings by jesting or putting interpersonal conflict in a wider context).
4. Eileen seemed to be effective at expressing group feelings (summarizing what those feelings were and describing the group's reactions to ideas or proposed solutions).
5. Mary participated in a variety of group maintenance functions. The checklist results would seem to indicate that Mary was a high participator.

Task Functions

These functions illustrate behaviors that are needed to complete the group's objectives. Many problem-solving tasks are essential to the successful completion of those objectives. For example, collecting data or seeking information, seeking and giving opinions, and summarizing and evaluating group decisions are essential group problem-solving tasks.

The Task Functions Observation Form shown in Exhibit 4C-2 is a checklist to help identify group members who are effective in task functions. The definitions of the functions to be observed follow (again, the numbers correspond to those listed in Exhibit 4C-2):

1. **Initiating:** proposing tasks or goals, defining a group problem, suggesting a procedure or ideas for solving a problem.

2. **Seeking Information:** requesting facts, seeking relevant information about group concerns.

3. **Giving Information:** offering facts, providing relevant information about group concerns.

4. **Seeking Opinion:** asking for expressions of feeling, requesting a statement or estimate, soliciting expressions of value, seeking suggestions and ideas.

5. **Giving Opinion:** stating a belief about a matter before the group, giving suggestions and ideas.

6. **Clarifying:** interpreting ideas or suggestions, clearing up confusions, defining terms, indicating alternatives and issues before the group.

7. **Elaborating:** giving examples, developing meanings, making generalizations, indicating how a proposal might work out if adopted.

8. **Summarizing:** pulling together related ideas, restating suggestions after group has discussed them, offering a decision or conclusion for the group to accept or reject.

9. **Coordinating:** showing relationships among various ideas or suggestions, trying to pull together ideas, suggestions, and activities of various subgroups or members.

10. **Evaluating:** submitting group decisions or accomplishments for comparison with group standards, measuring accomplishments against goals.

11. **Diagnosing:** determining sources of difficulties, ascertaining appropriate steps to take next, analyzing main blocks to progress.

Exhibit 4C-2 Task Functions Observation Checklist

Directions:
1. Observer should be familiar with the task functions as defined in the [accompanying] "Definition of Terms Used on Task Functions Observation Checklist."
2. Each member's name should be recorded in the space provided on the form.
3. Each time a group member performs a "Task Function," a slash or checkmark should be placed in the appropriate box.

Task Function	Group Members' Names				
	Edmund	*Pauline*	*Larry*	*Eileen*	*Mary*
1. Initiating		IIII		I	II
2. Seeking Information		III	IIII		II
3. Giving Information				IIII II	
			II	IIII	II
4. Seeking Opinion	IIII				
	III		I	I	II
5. Giving Opinion			III		IIII
6. Clarifying			II	I	IIII
7. Elaborating			I		IIII
8. Summarizing				I	III
9. Coordinating		IIII			IIII
10. Evaluating			IIII IIII IIII		I
11. Diagnosing			I		
12. Other					

Source: Adapted from J.W. Pfeiffer and J.E. Jones (eds.), *The 1972 Annual Handbook for Group Facilitators.* Contributed by Philip G. Hanson, V.A. Hospital, Houston, Tex. San Diego, Calif.: University Associates, 1972. Used with permission.

From the observations checked in Exhibit 4C-2, it may be concluded that:

1. Edmund did not participate in any group task functions.
2. Pauline was active in initiating (i.e., proposing tasks or defining a group problem), seeking information, seeking group members' opinions, and coordinating (i.e., showing relationships among various ideas or suggestions).

3. Larry was active in seeking information and evaluating the group's decisions.
4. Eileen was most active in giving information; she knew more than any other member of the group regarding the basic facts involved in the discussion.
5. Mary was the most active member of the group in involvement in task functions.

Nonfunctional Group Behaviors

Observation of these behaviors may help identify the group atmosphere: Do members work for status by criticizing or blaming others? Do they interfere with the ideas of others by rejecting them without consideration? Do they compete with each other rather than cooperate? Are any members withdrawn from the group?

Exhibit 4C-3 provides a checklist for identifying nonfunctional group behaviors. The definitions of the behaviors to be observed are in the following list (the terms keyed to the items in Exhibit 4C-3):

1. **Being Aggressive:** working for status by criticizing or blaming others, showing hostility against the group or some individual, deflating the ego or status of others.
2. **Blocking:** interfering with the progress of the group by going off on a tangent, citing personal experiences unrelated to the problem, arguing too much on a point, rejecting ideas without consideration.
3. **Self-Confessing:** using the group as a sounding board, expressing personal, nongroup-oriented feelings or points of view.
4. **Competing:** vying with others to produce the best idea, talking the most, playing the most roles, seeking to gain favor with the leader.
5. **Seeking Sympathy:** trying to induce other group members to be sympathetic to one's problems or misfortunes, deploring one's own situation, disparaging one's own ideas to gain support.
6. **Special Pleading:** introducing or supporting suggestions related to one's own pet concerns or philosophies, lobbying.
7. **Horsing Around:** clowning, joking, mimicking, disrupting the work of the group.
8. **Seeking Recognition:** attempting to call attention to one's self by loud or excessive talking, expressing extreme ideas, demonstrating unusual behavior.
9. **Withdrawal:** acting indifferent or passive, resorting to excessive formality, daydreaming, doodling, whispering to others, wandering from the subject.

Exhibit 4C-3 Nonfunctional Behavior Observation Checklist

Directions:
1. Observer should be familiar with the nonfunctional behaviors as defined in the [accompanying] list of "Nonfunctional Behavior Definitions."
2. Each member's name should be recorded in the space provided on the form.
3. Each time a group member performs a "Nonfunctional Behavior," a slash or check-mark should be placed in the appropriate box.

Nonfunctional Behavior	Group Members' Names				
	Edmund	*Pauline*	*Larry*	*Eileen*	*Mary*
1. Being Aggressive	IIII IIII IIII				
2. Blocking	IIII				
3. Self-Confessing	III				
4. Competing	IIII				II
5. Seeking Sympathy	I				
6. Special Pleading	I				
7. Horsing Around					
8. Seeking Recognition	IIII IIII				
9. Withdrawal					
10. Other					

Source: Adapted from J.W. Pfeiffer and J.E. Jones (eds.), *The 1972 Annual Handbook for Group Facilitators.* Contributed by Philip G. Hanson, V.A. Hospital, Houston, Tex. San Diego, Calif.: University Associates, 1972. Used with permission.

From the observations checked in Exhibit 4C-3, it may be concluded that:

1. Edmund was active in trying to block the objectives of the group. He was consistently aggressive, criticized and deflated the egos and status of others, blocked others' attempts at coming to solutions by rejecting ideas without giving them consideration. He constantly sought recognition by excessive talking and extreme ideas.
2. Pauline, Larry, and Eileen did not exhibit any nonfunctional group behaviors; only twice did Mary compete with others to gain favor with the leader.

Appendix 4-D

Rating Scale for Functional Level of Empathy

Source: Adapted from *Intervention in Human Services* (3rd ed.) by E.D. Schulman, published by The C.V. Mosby Company, St. Louis. Copyright © 1982, by permission of The C.V. Mosby Company. Scale adapted from "Dimensions of Therapists As Causal Factors in Therapeutic Change," by G.T. Barrett-Lennard in *Psychological Monograph 43:* 76, 1962; *Helping and Human Relations: A Primer for Lay and Professional Helpers* (Vols. I and II) by R.R. Carkhuff, published by Holt, Rinehart, & Winston, New York, 1969; and *Toward Effective Counseling and Psychotherapy* by C.B. Truax and R.R. Carkhuff, published by The Aldine Publishing Company, Chicago, 1967.

Unconditional Acceptance	*Positive Regard*	*Concrete Feedback*	*Developing Trust through Self-Exploration*
Level 1 Instructor actively offers student advice and is indifferent to student as a person. Often indicates that instructor knows what would be best for student and is actively critical. Instructor's overconcern for student interferes with open and clear discussion.	**Level 1** Instructor's verbal and nonverbal communication conveys a lack of appreciation for student. Instructor is more concerned with self. In fact, instructor may tell student more about own opinions and feelings (i.e., bragging), trying to increase own self-respect.	**Level 1** Instructor leads discussion or responds to student in an unclear, nonspecific, overintellectualized manner, avoiding personally significant situations or feelings.	**Level 1** Student mechanically talks about problems and feelings. Instructor fails to encourage student to produce personal and/or emotional material. Student, in effect, does not reveal self, either because of lack of encouragement from instructor or because student actively avoids discussing more personal concerns.
Level 2 Instructor ignores student, showing little interest or kindness. Instructor responds passively toward student considerably and is dependent on student's response.	**Level 2** Instructor's verbal and nonverbal expressions show lack of esteem for student. However, instructor's interest in and response to student is dependent on what student is talking about. At times instructor may respond with recognition of student's worth.	**Level 2** Instructor may talk about student's feelings and experiences but the discussion is unclear, intellectualized, and not sufficiently specific.	**Level 2** Student often responds mechanically, without exploring the meaning of experiences, and does not attempt to unveil or understand feelings. When instructor tries to encourage student to discuss personally relevant materials, student may agree or disagree, change the subject, or refuse to respond. Student does not produce new information related to own problems.

Unconditional Acceptance	Positive Regard	Concrete Feedback	Developing Trust through Self-Exploration
Level 3 Instructor communicates to student that student's feelings and behavior are important to instructor. Instructor claims responsibility for student and is semipossessive, telling client, "I want you to . . . ."	**Level 3** Instructor's verbal and nonverbal expressions indicate some degree of appreciation and esteem for student's feelings and experiences. Indicates that instructor values most of student's opinions and expressions about self.	**Level 3** At times instructor enables student to directly discuss more personally significant material clearly and concisely. In some areas of discussion, instructor does not assist student to be sufficiently specific.	**Level 3** Student willingly produces some personally relevant and new material but discusses it as if it has been rehearsed. Student shows some degree of feeling or spontaneity but often not both.
Level 4 Instructor shows deep commitment, interest, and concern for student's welfare. Accepts student as a person with little evaluation or criticism of student's beliefs or feelings.	**Level 4** Instructor's verbal and nonverbal expressions indicate appreciation for student's feelings. Instructor's responses enable student to feel worthwhile.	**Level 4** Instructor often helps student discuss personally significant feelings and experiences in specific and concise terms.	**Level 4** Student willingly introduces personally relevant and new material and discusses it openly, with emotional expressiveness. Student's verbal and nonverbal behaviors fit the feelings and information discussed. Instructor begins to help student get deeper into relationships with others (interpersonal), yet student is not fully enabled to discuss these relationships.
Level 5 Instructor shows unconditional acceptance of student as a person. Thus, student is free to be own self. Instructor shares student's hopes and successes as well as depressions and failures.	**Level 5** Instructor's verbal and nonverbal behaviors indicate deep esteem for student's problem solving. Instructor recognizes student as important to self and others.	**Level 5** Instructor enables student to freely discuss personally significant feelings and experiences in specific and concise terms, regardless of the emotions expressed.	**Level 5** Student is able to be, as well as to explore, self. Student actively and willingly engages in careful inward searching (intrapersonal) and discovers new views about self, feelings, and experiences.

SCORE SHEET FOR EMPATHY SCALE

Directions:

Place check under one of the levels for each characteristic. The Empathy Level equals the total number of checks under each category divided by 4, the total number of categories. This is the average level for all characteristics.

Example:

Unconditional acceptance	Level 2
Positive regard	Level 3
Concrete feedback	Level 2
Developing trust	Level 1

Total = 6

Divided by 3 = 2 (Level 2)

Levels

	1	2	3*	4	5
Unconditional acceptance					
Positive regard					
Concrete feedback					
Developing trust through self-exploration					
Total number of checks under each category					

*Minimum facilitative level.

Chapter 5

Instructional Revision

Those who refused to look through Galileo's telescope knew what they were about; if they did see the moons of Jupiter, then they would be forced to believe what they did not wish to believe. Therefore, it was wiser not to look.

John Ziman, 1966

Assessment of learning should not be an end in itself but rather an integral part of the instructional process. Through using evaluation results, educators continue what was effective and redevelop or discard what was ineffective.

How do educators know their efforts have been successful? Were the goals and objectives met? If they were met, were they appropriate? Were the learning activities worthwhile/successful/appropriate? Was it all worth the effort? Documenting the progress of an instructional program helps maintain some type of quality control.

Exhibit 5-1 again illustrates the systems model for instruction that was proposed in Chapter 2. As professionals practice their discipline, they also are held accountable for the quality of their activities. Unless they act to evaluate their instructional program, they cannot substantiate any claims that their efforts have made a difference. Perhaps more importantly, they do not have specific data with which to improve their efforts.

Exhibit 5-1 A Systems Model for Instruction

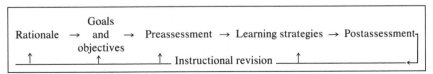

241

This chapter discusses why instructional programs are evaluated, offers a program evaluation model, suggests specific techniques for collecting and analyzing evaluative information, and looks at the use of the evaluation results for future program planning.

PROGRAM EVALUATION MODEL

The most important goal of program evaluation is to improve the nursing program for students. In addition it: (1) aids in future planning, (2) promotes informed decision making based on valid, reliable information, (3) contributes to the professional development of program personnel, and (4) ensures the accountability of expenditures in relation to costs and established objectives.

There is no shortage of references on program evaluation and/or evaluation models. However, this chapter is designed not to review this immense volume of literature but rather to take one evaluation model and suggest one possible route or blueprint for completing a program evaluation. This model focuses on the cumulative influence of the interaction of all the instructional components rather than on a specific course or program activity. It is concerned with changes in knowledges, skills, and attitudes as well as their impact on the individual. It involves how well the program satisfies the needs of both learners and employers.

Program evaluation thus includes not only instructional evaluation but also other dimensions. For example, results may indicate that all students have mastered the knowledges and skills needed for X but employer feedback may indicate that Y rather than X is necessary for nursing practice.

Stufflebeam, Foley, Gephart, Guba, Hammond, Merriman, and Provus (1971) offer a model for evaluation of instruction. The model includes four evaluation components: context, input, process, and product.

Evaluation of Context

Context evaluation helps answer the basic questions of where individuals are and what their needs are. It is done during the planning stage of the program to:

- define the environment in which the program will take place
- identify needs (i.e., student, community, personnel or staffing)
- identify and delineate constraints and problems underlying these needs.

Evaluation of Input

Input evaluation helps answer the basic question of how students will attain their objectives. The primary goal of input evaluation is to assess the capabilities of the instructional or training program to achieve its goals/objectives.

Input evaluation leads to the development of a plan for achieving the desired goals. The end product is an analysis of alternative procedural designs in terms of costs and benefits. For example, a staffing study completed during the context phase of the program evaluation may suggest that there is a shortage of nursing personnel.

The input evaluation should help answer a procedural design question in terms of costs/benefits: should the proposed program be designed for an associate, bachelor, or master's degree? These alternatives are assessed in terms of several relevant variables (e.g., available faculty, costs, and time). The resulting input evaluative information helps provide data and material needed for making decisions as to a choice of alternatives.

Evaluation of Process

Process evaluation helps answer the question of how students are doing in getting to their goals. It should help determine whether the program is being implemented as planned. Process evaluation should identify and monitor possible problems with such processes as methods and materials, faculty effectiveness, and the logistics of clinical education.

Evaluation of Product

Product evaluation helps answer the question of whether the goals have been reached. The primary objective is to determine the degree to which objectives and goals have been met and to relate this to context, input, and process information by determining the effectiveness of a program after it has been completed. While product evaluation traditionally has focused on assessing student accomplishment by such instruments as the Nursing Board Examination Score, student and employer surveys are suggested as additional, realistic, valid, and reliable measures of product. A program evaluation design should include a strong product evaluation component in addition to the assessment of context, input, and process.

The interdependency and interrelationships of these four components is important for making revisions to the instructional system. For example, if only product evaluation is conducted, the faculty might know whether the program was successful/unsuccessful but not be able to document why.

Context and input evaluation are crucial components in planning new programs. However, for operational programs the focus of evaluation efforts usually is at the process and product evaluation stages. The focus for the rest of this chapter is on techniques for operational process and product program evaluation.

TECHNIQUES FOR PROCESS EVALUATION

Sample evaluative questions that need to be asked to evaluate the process of the instructional program include:

- Were the instructional personnel effective?
- Were the teaching methods and instructional materials appropriate and effective?
- Were objectives met?
- Was the clinical education component well organized and effective?

Since the lack of specific techniques for collecting and analyzing process evaluation information has been a primary weakness of theoretical assessment models, this section suggests techniques for accumulating such material.

Measurement of Student Performance

The measurement of student performance probably is the most widely used process evaluation technique. It should focus on the competencies identified for practice. While many types of instruments can be used (e.g., paper-and-pencil achievement tests and clinical simulation examinations), specific student questionnaires also are valuable. Their results not only assess the competency attained by the students but also provide input for overall program evaluation and revision.

Table 5-1 is an example of a sample course evaluation form designed to gather process evaluation information. The form does not focus on traditional evaluation procedures for grading purposes but seeks instead to solicit input directly from students as to their perceptions of their accomplishments. As such it helps distinguish between program and instructional evaluation. The results also offer specific clues for making curricular revisions.

Table 5-1 Partial Course Evaluation Form

Pediatric Nursing Field Experience

Directions:
The following lists the major objectives that were identified for the pediatric nursing field experience. Using the following scales, please identify the extent to which you have achieved each objective (Achievement Scale) and your estimation of how confident you feel performing the objective (Confidence Scale):

1 = I have not achieved this objective.	1 = I do not feel confident.
2 = I have almost achieved this objective.	2 = I feel fairly confident about it.
3 = I have achieved this objective.	3 = I feel confident about it.

Objectives	Achievement Scale			Confidence Scale		
1. Assess the physical development of well children.	1	2	3	1	2	3
2. Assess the psychosocial development of well children.	1	2	3	1	2	3
3. Describe the variations of growth patterns in well children.	1	2	3	1	2	3
4. Complete a history taking.	1	2	3	1	2	3
5. Complete physical examinations.	1	2	3	1	2	3
6. Counsel parents in child-rearing practices.	1	2	3	1	2	3
7. Administer immunizations when appropriate.	1	2	3	1	2	3

Measurement of Faculty Effectiveness

Faculty effectiveness is one of the most important contributors to the success of a program. Traditionally, it has been evaluated by observation and rating by a supervisor and by peers, rating by students, and self-observation via videotapes. However, ratings by students not only are widely used but also have created much controversy.

For purposes of this discussion, the evaluation of faculty is not to judge the adequacy of individuals nor to recommend continue/not continue but to provide feedback for strengthening the instructors' effectiveness, thereby improving the nursing program. Determining faculty effectiveness is an interdependent part of curriculum improvement activities. The primary goal is to produce information that will help make the program better—to improve teaching/learning in reference to objectives. All else is secondary to this central goal.

The primary approach to evaluation of instruction often involves rating forms developed for use by students. However, the instructional role is much broader. There are several other tasks/roles/decisions that should be considered in assessing faculty effectiveness. These include the evaluation of the nonteaching aspects of instruction:

- assessing the faculty advisory role
- assessing continuing scholarship
- assessing the planning for instruction (i.e., course objectives, syllabuses, selection of experiences to meet course objectives, appropriate assignments, development of classroom tests, etc.).

Each of these approaches to evaluating faculty effectiveness is discussed next.

THE STUDENT RATING FORM

For student evaluation of faculty to be effective, some basic assumptions should be agreed upon:

- A mutual feeling of trust must have been developed between students and teacher.
- The information must be used solely for the improvement of instruction and not for determining salary, tenure, or promotion.
- The evaluation instrument must have been developed by or accepted by the teacher.
- Results must be confidential and collected by the individual instructor, who alone should make the decision as to whether or not to share the outcome with others.

One of the primary advantages of student evaluation is that it offers instructors the opportunity to receive feedback about their "blind self." For example, they may believe they are sensitive listeners yet in reality may regularly interrupt students. Student-teacher exchanges about what was planned and what actually happened can improve instructor effectiveness. The "Johari Window" in Figure 5-1 helps illustrate the relationships between what an instructor believes is being done (i.e., one's espoused theory) and what actually is occurring (i.e., one's theory in use) (Luft, 1969). Johari window is a graphic model revealing the degree of openness of oneself. Joseph Luft (1969) developed the concept with Harry Ingham.

Figure 5-1 Johari Window's Relationship to Evaluation of Teaching

	What the students know about the teacher	What the students do not know about the teacher	
What the teacher knows about self	Public or Open Self 1	Secret or Hidden Self 2	
What the teacher does not know about self	Blind Self 3	Undiscovered or Subconscious Self 4	Aspects of teacher behavior not known to teacher or student

Johari was derived from a combination of their first names—Joseph and Harry.

Cell 1 of Figure 5-1, the public or open self, contains common information known about the teacher by both students and instructor. This is the area where communication is very effective. As the teacher receives information from the students about effectiveness, this area enlarges.

Cell 2, the secret or hidden self, contains information the instructor knows about self, teaching, and professional behavior that the students do not know. In a humanistic teaching environment, the size of this cell is reduced because individuals share more information about themselves with each other. Consequently the hidden self is diminished.

Cell 3, the blind self, contains information about the teacher's behavior that is known to the students but not to the instructor. For example, the teacher may have a self-concept of being fair but in reality have several "teacher's pets." Student evaluation of faculty can assist in reducing the blind self.

Cell 4, the undiscovered or subconscious self, contains aspects of teacher behavior not known to either teacher or student. For example, regarding subconscious motivations and feelings, a young woman may marry a much older man because she believes she truly loves him, but in reality she is subconsciously searching for a father she never had.

Appropriately used, faculty evaluation by students can help reduce the teacher's hidden and blind self and increase the open self. Instructors who are truly interested in improving their competence are likely to seek and utilize feedback from their students. Clearly this is process or formative evaluation.

Faculty members usually require that the items on any student evaluation form be appropriate or specific to the discipline and their personal conception of "good teaching." Consequently, many instructors seek to develop their own evaluation instrument or to assist in the development of the student one. The extensive discussion as faculty members either develop or adapt existing student evaluation forms probably has some positive indirect impact on the quality of teaching.

Many evaluation forms are available for students, most of them rating scales. However, if the instructor is opposed to a rating scale, the students may use open-ended essay or short-answer questions.

The author has adopted the evaluation forms developed after extensive research by Hildebrand, Wilson, and Dienst (1971). A brief description of the research, including a sample of the revised student evaluation form, is presented next.

Sample Teacher Evaluation Form

After extensive research, Hildebrand et al. (1971) developed two instruments for evaluating teaching—the *Student Description of Teachers* and the *Colleague Description of Teachers*. These scales provide a profile of individual instructor behavior as perceived by students or colleagues. The research identifies five components as comprising teaching effectiveness. They are illustrated in Exhibit 5-2.

Exhibit 5-2 Characteristics of Teacher Effectiveness

Instructor Knowledge (Analytic/ Synthetic Approach)	Organization and Clarity of Presentation	Instructor-Group Interaction	Instructor-Individual Interaction	Dynamism and Enthusiasm

1. *Analytic/Synthetic Approach:* The instructor has command of the subject, presents material in an analytic way, contrasts various points of view, discusses current developments, and relates topics to other areas of knowledge.
2. *Organization and Clarity:* The instructor makes self clear, states objectives, summarizes major points, presents material in an organized manner, and provides examples.
3. *Instructor-Group Interaction:* The instructor is sensitive to the response of the class, encourages student participation, and welcomes questions and discussion.
4. *Instructor-Individual Student Interaction:* The instructor is available to and friendly toward students, is interested in them as individuals, is respected as a person, and is valued for advice not directly related to the course.
5. *Dynamism/Enthusiasm:* The instructor enjoys teaching, is enthusiastic about the subject, makes the course exciting, and has self-confidence.

An adaptation of the evaluation form is illustrated in Table 5-2. Items 1 to 4 measure the instructor's analytic/synthetic approach; items 5 to 10, organization/clarity; items 11 to 15, instructor/group interaction; items 16 to 19, instructor/individual interaction; and items 20 to 24 the instructor's dynamism/enthusiasm. This is a medium-length form. Obviously, additional items can be added, and it can be adapted as desired. For example, the following items were found to be descriptive of teachers of small classes and may be used by the instructor to modify the questionnaire for seminars, small classes, and/or the laboratory setting:

1. Discusses practical applications.
2. Makes difficult topics easy to understand.
3. Gives examinations requiring creative, original thinking.
4. Knows when students are bored or confused.
5. Keeps well informed about the progress of the class.
6. Reminds students to see the instructor if they are having difficulty.
7. Encourages students to express feelings and opinions.
8. Provides time for discussion and questions.
9. Grasps quickly what a student is asking or telling.
10. Informs students of events related to the course.

While the results can be used for several purposes (i.e., faculty development, promotion, tenure, merit pay) it is suggested that they be utilized primarily by individual instructors to analyze and evaluate their own teaching. As such, instructors distribute the instrument to their own classes and use the results to learn more about the students' perception of their teaching.

There has been much criticism of student evaluation of faculty. Critics content that it (1) does little general good and may do some harm, (2) may create competition among faculty members, (3) has the potential for becoming formalized and rigid, (4) may furnish inadequate or misleading information, (5) is influenced by too many other variables (e.g., personality of instructor, workload, difficulty of course), and (6) is an invasion of privacy. In addition, some faculty members believe that students are not capable of evaluating instruction.

Extensive research has challenged much of this criticism. Rosenshine, Cohen, and Furst (1973), in a study of seven student variables in 1,200 college classes, report that there is no significant relationship between student ratings and year in school, grade point average, expected grade, age, number of previous courses in field, sex, and marital status. Other studies are not unanimous with regard to expected grade.

Table 5-2 Teacher Evaluation Form

Instructor _____

Directions:
Please circle your response to each of the following statements as they relate to your instructor.

5 = Strongly Agree
4 = Agree
3 = Undecided
2 = Disagree
1 = Strongly Disagree
0 = Doesn't Apply or Don't Know

	SA	A	U	D	SD	DA
1. Discusses points of view other than own, if appropriate to the specific class.	5	4	3	2	1	0
2. Contrasts implications of various theories, if appropriate to the specific class.	5	4	3	2	1	0
3. Discusses recent developments in the field.	5	4	3	2	1	0
4. Presents origins of ideas and concepts.	5	4	3	2	1	0
5. Explains clearly.	5	4	3	2	1	0
6. Is well prepared.	5	4	3	2	1	0
7. Conducts class in an organized fashion.	5	4	3	2	1	0
8. Is careful and precise in answering questions.	5	4	3	2	1	0
9. Summarizes majòr points.	5	4	3	2	1	0
10. States objectives for class sessions.	5	4	3	2	1	0
11. Encourages class participation.	5	4	3	2	1	0
12. Invites students to share their knowledge and experiences.	5	4	3	2	1	0
13. Invites criticism of own ideas.	5	4	3	2	1	0
14. Knows whether or not the class understands the instructor.	5	4	3	2	1	0
15. Has students apply concepts to demonstrate understanding.	5	4	3	2	1	0
16. Has genuine interest in students.	5	4	3	2	1	0
17. Is friendly toward students.	5	4	3	2	1	0
18. Relates to students as individuals.	5	4	3	2	1	0
19. Respects students as persons.	5	4	3	2	1	0
20. Is a dynamic and energetic person.	5	4	3	2	1	0
21. Has interesting style of presentation.	5	4	3	2	1	0
22. Seems to enjoy teaching.	5	4	3	2	1	0
23. Is enthusiastic about class subject.	5	4	3	2	1	0
24. Seems to have self-confidence.	5	4	3	2	1	0

Additional Comments Are Welcome.

Source: Adapted from *Evaluating University Teaching* by M. Hildebrand, Robert C. Wilson, and E.R. Dienst, published by the University of California, Center for Research and Development in Higher Education, Berkeley, Calif. Copyright © 1971, by permission of the author.

Class size has been shown to have a relationship to ratings (Menges, 1973). To counteract this bias, separate norms for small, medium, and large classes should be considered. This same bias is true for required vs. elective courses. Furthermore, other things being equal, in addition to smaller classes' being more effective, discussions are more effective than lectures, and student-centered discussions are more effective than instructor-centered ones in promoting retention, application, problem solving, attitude change, and motivation for further study (Dressel, 1978).

The research seems to support the following statements:

1. Teaching effectiveness and scholarly publication are unrelated to each other (Costin, Greenough, & Menges, 1971; Siegfried & White, 1973).
2. Administrators' ratings of teachers are interchangeable with ratings by colleagues.
3. Ratings by colleagues agree fairly well with those by students.
4. There is a very small correlation between self-evaluation and assessments by administrators and students (Blackburn & Clark, 1975).

ASSESSING FACULTY ADVISORY ROLE

Faculty advising receives far less attention than instruction yet it is very important to student learning. Faculty advisers should regard students first as individuals with specific needs, aspirations, and interests and second as department majors. For example, if during advisement it appears clear that a career in nursing is not for a student, the faculty should help the individual explore other career alternatives. To do this adequately, the faculty needs in-depth knowledge about the institution, its course offerings, and its regulations. For faculty members to perceive advising as a valued function they must have time to prepare for it and must be adequately rewarded for it.

The following questions may suggest items for developing a process for evaluating the effectiveness of faculty advising (Dressel, 1978):

1. Are students satisfied with the advising they receive (including help in course selection in reference to a vocation)?
2. Are degree requirements being met without loss of time?
3. Are individual adaptations (including transfer of credit, waiver of requirements, and variation in program) justified on the basis of educational principles allowed?

4. How frequently do advisers refer students to other appropriate services (e.g., personal and vocational counseling, learning center)?
5. Is the advisement function appropriately recognized and rewarded?

Evidence of continuing scholarship is essential for all nurse educators.
The traditional view of continuing scholarship is evidence of a research
and publication record. However, an essential factor is that the nurse
educator remain up to date with practice, which means continuing, systematic, planned experience in the clinical setting.

Nurse educators should maintain contact with the clinical setting and
with real patients. If nursing faculty members do not know what is happening in the field, they will not be as effective as teachers. Furthermore,
their students may graduate without the necessary current skills for safe,
effective practice. Planning for these experiences may be difficult to sched-
ule and may be met with resistance from some instructors. However, if
done successfully, the up-to-date clinical experience will immensely enrich
the teaching/learning environment. Consequently, continuing scholarship
can be evaluated in part by documenting how individuals maintain their
links with clinical practice.

Secondary measures of continuing scholarship can be assessed by examining the textbooks and materials used to complement instruction. How
recent are the items listed in the bibliography? Indeed, is a bibliography
(or references) provided?

Obviously, involvement in research and publication is the most traditional measure of continuing scholarship yet an equally important gauge
is continued active involvement in clinical practice.

ASSESSING INSTRUCTIONAL PLANNING

Evaluating the selection of educational materials and methods is another
important faculty responsibility. This expands the teacher's role beyond
that of a mere dispenser of information to the broader scope of a planner
and evaluator of the educational process. When materials and methods
are thoughtfully chosen, developed, and/or adapted, they contribute to a
quality educational experience. Table 5-3 is an example of a form for
evaluating textbook and supplemental reading materials.

Evaluating the development of classroom tests also is an important
faculty function. Is there congruence between the class objectives and the
test items? Are multiple-choice and essay items used appropriately? Are
clinical simulation examinations used for clinical learning? Are the tests

Table 5-3 Textbook and Supplemental Reading Evaluation

Subject _____ ___ _____
Title of Book __ ... _____
Copyright Date _____ Author(s) _____
Publisher _____
Evaluator _____

Directions:
Please evaluate the textbook or supplemental reading material using the following scale:

1 = Yes
2 = No
3 = Somewhat
4 = Impossible to tell

Objectives:
1. Does the title indicate the content of the reading material?   1   2   3   4
2. Does the reading material require students to use higher cognitive skills?   1   2   3   4
3. Does the reading material complement the goals and objectives of the course?   1   2   3   4

Content:
4. Does the reading material develop accurate concepts and generalizations?   1   2   3   4
5. Does the reading material require students to employ rational thought in discovering and testing value positions?   1   2   3   4
6. Would you recommend this reading material?   1   2   3   4
7. Is the content of the reading material appropriate to the abilities and needs of the students using it?   1   2   3   4
8. Are historical, social, and scientific discussions based on the most current evidence?   1   2   3   4
9. How would you rank this reading material among those reviewed?
    1st choice
    2nd choice
    3rd choice
    4th choice
    5th choice
10. How would you compare this reading material with existing materials?
    Better
    About the same
    Worse
11. Would you use the textbook or supplemental reading material in your own class?
    Yes _____
    No _____ (Please explain)

valid and reliable? Are students encouraged to view evaluation as a way to improve their performance?

An indispensable part of learning is the recognition and admission of error combined with the ability to profit from mistakes. Failure must be regarded as a challenge, not as a disabling and uncorrectable event that inhibits further progress. The faculty member who treats failure otherwise is not teaching but merely is rewarding those who are capable of progressing without assistance (Dressel, 1978). Many clinical nursing procedures are sufficiently complex to require much practice. Is this practice time available in the faculty's planning for instruction?

This discussion of the evaluation of instruction has focused on its primary purpose: to improve teaching/learning in reference to classroom objectives. Because evaluation is a complex process, no one method by itself is adequate. Various facets of the teaching/learning process can be examined by different means. Some methods of evaluating faculty effectiveness have been discussed—students' rating of teachers, assessing the faculty advising role, looking at continuing scholarship, and appraising the planning for instruction. While additional methods exist—such as self-appraisal through the use of audiotapes and/or videotapes and colleague evaluation—they are not analyzed here.

Many nurses as professional clinicians are not prepared for college teaching, for advisement, or for many of the other tasks to which a large amount of their time is committed. As a result, the institution has the responsibility to provide inservice education. Just as instructors should not evaluate students on objectives that were not covered in the teaching/learning process, neither should teachers be evaluated on activities for which they have had no formal preparation.

TECHNIQUES FOR PRODUCT EVALUATION

The most common method of determining program effectiveness is the percentage of graduates passing the nursing board examination. However, the employer survey and follow-up of former learners can offer additional useful information.

The Employer Survey

The primary objective of the employer survey (see Appendix 5-A) is to assess the performance of former students, thereby contributing to the evaluation of the instructional program. Related and/or secondary objectives are (1) to elicit employers' recommendations for improving the program, (2) to determine their recruitment practices, and (3) to contribute to improved public relations between them and the educational programs.

For purposes of this discussion, the basic function of an employer survey is to answer the questions, "How did the graduates of the nursing program perform on the job? Were the cognitive, psychomotor, and affective objectives of the curriculum met?"

This discussion is not designed to provide instruction on the development of an employer follow-up form but rather to encourage the use of follow-up studies as a component of product evaluation. Appendix 5-B is an example of a student follow-up survey that is strongly linked to the program objectives.

There must be congruence between program objectives and evaluation. Without this strong link, the faculty will not know what part of the teaching/learning sequence to change to improve the program. Employer feedback that is specifically related to program objectives will provide specific information for making improvements.

The Student Follow-Up Study

A student follow-up study is much broader than a statistical placement report and may include dropouts as well as graduates. Follow-up studies designed to evaluate the effectiveness of the instruction can provide important feedback regarding the strengths and weaknesses of the program as perceived by students.

Student follow-up studies may have more than one objective. For example, in addition to evaluating the effectiveness of the instructional program, they may be simultaneously designed to:

- Determine career patterns of former students: Follow-up studies at one-, three-, and five-year intervals can provide useful information regarding such patterns.
- Determine immediate demand for nursing positions: A follow-up survey can provide information on the types of jobs students are getting when they graduate. This may have direct impact on curricular revision. For example, if 75 percent of the graduates find employment in long-term care facilities, this may affect curriculum emphasis.
- Determine mobility of graduates: A program designed to prepare individuals for the community that produces a large percentage of graduates who cannot find local employment would indicate the local job market may be saturated. Depending upon the mission of the program, admissions may be reduced.

Developing the Follow-Up Study

The purpose and objectives of the follow-up study must be established before anything else is done. First, the overall goal must be determined, then specific objectives formulated. For example:

Overall Goal:
- To determine the adequacy of the bachelor degree nursing program to prepare individuals for entry level positions.

Specific Objectives:
- To determine whether program objectives are consistent with entry level job requirements.
- To identify program strengths and weaknesses.
- To determine whether students are entering jobs for which they were prepared.
- To determine whether students who complete the program have the necessary cognitive, psychomotor, and affective skills to perform as entry level nurses.

While the very detailed student follow-up questionnaire illustrated in Appendix 5-B may be appropriate for a six-month to one-year alumni follow-up study, if much more time passes students will have had such a variety of new experiences that their recollection of specific courses/objectives/accomplishments may not be accurate. A more generalized questionnaire may be appropriate for a three-year or five-year graduate follow-up study (see the follow-up study questionnaire illustrated in Appendix 5-C).

USING RESULTS TO ENCOURAGE CHANGE

Nursing educators must remember that no matter how well managed or how appropriate recommended curricular changes, there always will be some resistance to change. For change means altering or giving up part or all of a previously held value, concept, belief, attitude, or behavior. Change is easier to influence if the entire faculty has been involved in the total evaluation process. When everyone is involved, the faculty members share not only ownership but also responsibility for the program; the needs and feelings of all are viewed as important. Since successful implementation of the recommendations requires the commitment, cooperation, and support of the faculty, all of its members must be meaningfully involved in the process.

Stufflebeam's (1971) model provides a systematic approach to evaluation. The model broadens the scope of assessment. It provides a mechanism for a systematic information-gathering system and for both formative and summative evaluation. It requires staff members to become sensitive to the many internal and external factors affecting the success of a program. As the evaluation information is used to revise the operation, it helps ensure the possibility that the nursing program will remain strong and viable.

REFERENCES

Blackburn, R.T., & Clark, M.J. An assessment of faculty performance: Some correlates between administrator, colleague, student, and self-ratings. *Sociology of Education,* 1975, *48,* 242–256.

Costin, F.; Greenough, W.T.; & Menges, R.J. Student ratings of college teaching: Reliability, validity, and usefulness. *Review of Educational Research,* 1971, *41,* 511–535.

Dressel, P.L. *Handbook of academic evaluation.* San Francisco: Jossey-Bass, Inc., Publishers, 1978.

Haase, P.T. A proposed system for nursing: Theoretical framework (Pt. 2). Atlanta, Ga.: Southern Regional Educational Board, 1976.

Hildebrand, M.; Wilson, R.C.; & Dienst, E.R. *Evaluating university teaching.* Berkeley, Calif.: University of California, Center for Research and Development in Higher Education, 1971.

Luft, J. *Of human interaction.* New York: National Press Books, 1969.

Menges, R.J. The new reporters: Students rate instruction. Evaluating learning and teaching, C.R. Pace (ed.), *New Directions for Higher Education,* No. 4, Winter 1973.

Rosenshine, B.; Cohen, A.; & Furst, N. Correlates of student preference ratings. *Journal of College Student Personnel,* 1973, *14,* 269–272.

Siegfried, J.J., & White, K.J. Teaching and publishing as determinants of academic salaries. *Journal of Economic Education,* 1973, *4,* 90–99.

Stufflebeam, D.I.; Foley, W.J.; Gephart, W.J.; Guba, E.G.; Hammond, R.I.; Merriman, H.O.; & Provus, M.M. *Educational evaluation and decision making.* Itasca, Ill.: F.E. Peacock, Publishers, Inc., 1971.

Appendix 5-A

Sample Employer Questionnaire

Name of Person Being Evaluated _____

Present Title _____ Department _____

(If any of the above information is incorrect, please make the necessary corrections.)

Relation of Evaluation to Individual Being Evaluated (Please check one)

_____ Head Nurse

_____ Supervisor

_____ Other (Please Specify)

Please check the item that most accurately describes your relationship with the person being evaluated.

_____ Direct Supervision   _____ Frequent Contact

_____ Indirect Supervision   _____ Occasional Contact

Directions:

For each item, please check the column that indicates your evaluation of the individual's performance. Each item describes one of the objectives for our nursing program. Use the following scale:*

1 = Is Not Competent
2 = Is Somewhat Competent
3 = Is Competent
4 = Is Very Competent
0 = Not Observed

   1. Recognizes behavioral, physiological, and envi-   1   2   3   4   0
      ronmental cues related to nursing care.

---

*Competency statements adapted from *A Proposed System for Nursing: Theoretical Framework,* Part 2, by Patricia T. Haase, published by Southern Regional Education Board, Atlanta, Ga. pp. 75–107. Copyright © 1976, by permission of Southern Regional Education Board.

2. Uses units of information to analyze and interpret data, to recognize patterns and relationships, and to predict outcomes.   1 2 3 4 0

3. Makes inferences using problem-solving methods.   1 2 3 4 0

4. Evaluates data by appraising, assessing, or criticizing on the basis of criteria, norms, or desired outcomes.   1 2 3 4 0

5. Develops new remedies, action plans, or hypotheses, including creating, originating, and integrating ideas and proposals that are new.   1 2 3 4 0

6. Demonstrates mutual and reciprocal interpersonal working relationships.   1 2 3 4 0

7. Demonstrates empathy and acceptance of others' behavior.   1 2 3 4 0

8. Strives for objectivity in working with clients.   1 2 3 4 0

9. Maintains adaptability and flexibility in working with clients.   1 2 3 4 0

10. Develops and maintains social consciousness.   1 2 3 4 0

11. Demonstrates warmth, concern, and respect for client.   1 2 3 4 0

12. Respects client's life choices (does not impose own value system).   1 2 3 4 0

13. Demonstrates unconditional positive regard for client.   1 2 3 4 0

14. Focuses on others (expresses interest, offers assistance, shows concern and interest that may be interpreted as warmth, caring, respect: introduces self, calls client by name, looks directly at client, touches, listens, responds to questions, maintains availability).   1 2 3 4 0

15. Respects and maintains self-boundaries (recognizes own feelings and beliefs and distinguishes them from client's feelings and beliefs).   1 2 3 4 0

16. Accepts negative feelings from clients.   1 2 3 4 0

17. Nurtures client by comforting, consoling, and sharing.   1 2 3 4 0

18. Manipulates and controls client's environment to provide maximum comfort (e.g., noise, temperature, bed linens, accessories).   1 2 3 4 0

19. Maintains and restores hygiene of skin, mucous membranes, and appendages.   1 2 3 4 0

20. Provides basic hygiene for care of intact skin   1 2 3 4 0
and simple prostheses (eyeglasses and den-
tures).
21. Provides advanced hygiene care of decubiti,   1 2 3 4 0
ostomies, and braces.
22. Protects client against infection by applying   1 2 3 4 0
aseptic techniques and by the proper use, care,
and disinfection of equipment.
23. Prepares, administers, and monitors nutritional   1 2 3 4 0
and fluid intake.
24. Describes attributes of fluid, excretory, and   1 2 3 4 0
secretory losses accurately.
25. Provides for secretion-excretion removal by   1 2 3 4 0
competently applying the following methods:
   a. Basic: oral, pharyngeal, suction, enemas   1 2 3 4 0
   b. Advanced: clapping and percussive respi-   1 2 3 4 0
     ratory techniques
   c. Tracheal suctioning   1 2 3 4 0
   d. Catheterization   1 2 3 4 0
   e. Gastric aspiration   1 2 3 4 0
26. Establishes and maintains drainage systems:
   a. Simple: e.g., humidifiers, nebulizers, Iso-   1 2 3 4 0
     lettes
   b. Complex: e.g., Bourne, Emerson   1 2 3 4 0
27. Records client data accurately.   1 2 3 4 0
28. Aids in diagnosis by obtaining specimens.   1 2 3 4 0
29. Performs physical exam: 1 2 3 4 0
   a. Basic: vital signs, "basic" observations   1 2 3 4 0
     (cyanosis, consciousness)
   b. Intermediate: palpation, percussion, aus-   1 2 3 4 0
     cultation
   c. Advanced: vaginals, pelvics, rectals   1 2 3 4 0
30. Prepares and administers medications compe-   1 2 3 4 0
tently.
31. Provides dressing and wound care
   a. Basic: Band-Aid   1 2 3 4 0
   b. Advanced: burn dressing   1 2 3 4 0
32. Applies support devices and braces
   a. Basic: elastic stocking   1 2 3 4 0
   b. Advanced: splinting, traction   1 2 3 4 0
33. Maintains total systems
   a. Basic: Foley care   1 2 3 4 0

    b. Advanced: ensure patency of chest tubes   1 2 3 4 0
34. Performs basic resuscitative measures
    a. Artificial respiration, external cardiac mas-   1 2 3 4 0
       sage

Would you consider another graduate from our program if you had an available position?   _____ 1. Yes
                                            _____ 2. No

    Comments:

Do you see any observable difference between our former student and other new bachelor degree nursing students you hire?   _____ 1. Yes
                                              _____ 2. No

    Comments:

We would appreciate any additional comments you may have that would assist us in improving our nursing program.

Appendix 5-B

Sample Student Follow-Up Questionnaire

1. _____
    Last Name   First Name   Middle Name

2. _____
    Present Address: Street & Number   Post Office   State   Zip

3. Telephone: (Home) _____ (Business) _____

4. Present Position _____

_____
Employer's Name   Address: Street & Number   Post Office   State   Zip

5. Present gross annual salary. $ _____

Directions:
The following list represents the major objectives of your nursing program. For each item, please indicate the extent to which you feel confident doing the skill and your estimation of how important it is in the performance of your job. Use the following scales:*

Competence	*Importance*
1 = I do not feel competent	1 = Not important
2 = I feel somewhat competent	2 = Somewhat important
3 = I feel competent	3 = Important
4 = I feel very competent	4 = Very important

---

*Competency statements adapted from *A Proposed System for Nursing: Theoretical Framework,* Part 2, by Patricia T. Haase, published by Southern Regional Education Board, Atlanta, Ga. pp. 75–107. Copyright © 1976, by permission of Southern Regional Education Board.

	Competence	Importance
1. Recognizes behavioral, physiological, and environmental cues related to nursing care.	1 2 3 4	1 2 3 4
2. Uses units of information to analyze and interpret data, to recognize patterns and relationships, and to predict outcomes.	1 2 3 4	1 2 3 4
3. Makes inferences using problem-solving methods.	1 2 3 4	1 2 3 4
4. Evaluates data by appraising, assessing, or criticizing on the basis of criteria, norms, or desired outcomes.	1 2 3 4	1 2 3 4
5. Develops new remedies, action plans, or hypotheses, including creating, originating, and integrating ideas and proposals that are new.	1 2 3 4	1 2 3 4
6. Demonstrates mutual and reciprocal interpersonal working relationships.	1 2 3 4	1 2 3 4
7. Demonstrates empathy and acceptance of others' behavior.	1 2 3 4	1 2 3 4
8. Strives for objectivity in working with clients.	1 2 3 4	1 2 3 4
9. Maintains adaptability and flexibility in working with clients.	1 2 3 4	1 2 3 4
10. Develops and maintains social consciousness.	1 2 3 4	1 2 3 4
11. Demonstrates warmth, concern, and respect for client.	1 2 3 4	1 2 3 4
12. Respects client's life choices (does not impose own value system).	1 2 3 4	1 2 3 4
13. Demonstrates unconditional positive regard for client.	1 2 3 4	1 2 3 4
14. Focuses on others (expresses interest, offers assistance, shows concern and interest that may be interpreted as warmth, caring, respect).	1 2 3 4	1 2 3 4

	Competence	Importance
15. Respects and maintains self-boundaries (recognizes own feelings and beliefs and distinguishes them from client's feelings and beliefs).	1 2 3 4	1 2 3 4
16. Accepts negative feelings from clients.	1 2 3 4	1 2 3 4
17. Nurtures client by comforting, consoling, and sharing.	1 2 3 4	1 2 3 4
18. Manipulates and controls client's environment to provide maximum comfort (e.g., noise, temperature, bed linens, accessories).	1 2 3 4	1 2 3 4
19. Maintains and restores hygiene of skin, mucous membranes, and appendages.	1 2 3 4	1 2 3 4
20. Provides basic hygiene for care of intact skin and simple prostheses (eyeglasses and dentures).	1 2 3 4	1 2 3 4
21. Provides advanced hygiene care of decubiti, ostomies, and braces.	1 2 3 4	1 2 3 4
22. Protects client against infection by applying aseptic techniques and by the proper use, care, and disinfection of equipment.	1 2 3 4	1 2 3 4
23. Prepares, administers, and monitors nutritional and fluid intake.	1 2 3 4	1 2 3 4
24. Describes attributes of fluid, excretory, and secretory losses accurately.	1 2 3 4	1 2 3 4
25. Provides for secretion-excretion removal by competently applying the following methods:		
a. Basic: oral, pharyngeal, suction, enemas	1 2 3 4	1 2 3 4
b. Advanced: clapping and percussive respiratory techniques	1 2 3 4	1 2 3 4

	Competence	Importance
c. Tracheal suctioning	1 2 3 4	1 2 3 4
d. Catheterization	1 2 3 4	1 2 3 4
e. Gastric aspiration	1 2 3 4	1 2 3 4
26. Establishes and maintains drainage systems:		
a. Simple: e.g., humidifiers, nebulizers, Isolettes	1 2 3 4	1 2 3 4
b. Complex: e.g., Bourne, Emerson	1 2 3 4	1 2 3 4
27. Records client data accurately.	1 2 3 4	1 2 3 4
28. Aids in diagnosis by obtaining specimens.	1 2 3 4	1 2 3 4
29. Performs physical exam:		
a. Basic: vital signs, "basic" observations (cyanosis, consciousness)	1 2 3 4	1 2 3 4
b. Intermediate: palpation, percussion, auscultation	1 2 3 4	1 2 3 4
c. Advanced: vaginals, pelvics, rectals	1 2 3 4	1 2 3 4
30. Prepares and administers medications competently.	1 2 3 4	1 2 3 4
31. Provides dressing and wound care		
a. Basic: Band-Aid	1 2 3 4	1 2 3 4
b. Advanced: burn dressing	1 2 3 4	1 2 3 4
32. Applies support devices and braces		
a. Basic: elastic stocking	1 2 3 4	1 2 3 4
b. Advanced: splinting, traction	1 2 3 4	1 2 3 4
33. Maintains total systems		
a. Basic: Foley care	1 2 3 4	1 2 3 4
b. Advanced: ensure patency of chest tubes	1 2 3 4	1 2 3 4
34. Performs basic resuscitative measures		
a. Artificial respiration, external cardiac massage	1 2 3 4	1 2 3 4

Name of Employer for Evaluation
Please indicate the name of the individual to whom you gave the Employer Evaluation Form in the event we have to follow up if it is not returned.

_____

Name   Address

Thank you for all your time and effort.

Appendix 5-C

3-Year or 5-Year Graduate Follow-Up Questionnaire

I.   What is your present status? (Mark all that apply to you.)

    1. Employed full time in nursing or related field
    2. Employed part time in nursing or related field
    3. Unemployed and looking for work
    4. Unemployed and not looking for work
    5. Full-time homemaker
    6. In military service
    7. Continuing school full time
    8. Continuing school part time
        School _____
        City and State _____
    9. Other (please specify) _____

II. How would you describe the relationship between your present job and your nursing program at _____ (name of institution)?

    1. Program directly related to job
    2. Program somewhat related to job
    3. Program only slightly related to job
    4. Program not at all related to job

III. If you marked No. 4 above, what factors influenced your decision to take a job unrelated to your program?

    1. Unable to get a related job
    2. Not willing to leave this area
    3. Higher salary

4. Self-satisfaction
5. Decided to enter another field for other reasons
6. Other, please specify _____

IV. If you are in nursing, in which of the following areas are you now working?

___ 1. Direct patient care
___ 2. Supervisor of patient care
___ 3. Administration of patient care
___ 4. Teaching (nursing related)
___ 5. Research (nursing related)
___ 6. Other (Please specify) _____

V. Are you currently enrolled in an educational institution for degree credit?

___ 1. Yes
___ 2. No
If yes, what degree are you working toward? _____

VI. How important for your educational development have the following experiences been?

0 = Not Applicable
1 = Not Important
2 = Little Importance
3 = Somewhat Important
4 = Important
5 = Very Important

1. Lecture courses in major field	0	1	2	3	4	5
2. Seminar courses in major field	0	1	2	3	4	5
3. Clinical experiences in major field	0	1	2	3	4	5
4. Interdisciplinary courses	0	1	2	3	4	5
5. Independent study courses	0	1	2	3	4	5
6. Informal interaction with faculty	0	1	2	3	4	5
7. Informal interaction with other students	0	1	2	3	4	5
8. Classroom teaching strategies						
Lecture/discussions	0	1	2	3	4	5
Discussions	0	1	2	3	4	5
Role playing	0	1	2	3	4	5

Use of case studies   0 1 2 3 4 5
Community field work   0 1 2 3 4 5

VII. Please rate the quality of instruction for the following courses in your nursing program and your estimation of how important each course was to your performance on the job. Use the following scales:

Quality	*Importance*
1 = Minimum level	1 = Not important
2 = Below average	2 = Somewhat important
3 = Average	3 = Important
4 = Above average	
5 = Superior	
0 = Doesn't apply or don't know	

	Quality of Instruction						*Importance*		
1. Biology of disease	1	2	3	4	5	0	1	2	3
2. Nursing assessment	1	2	3	4	5	0	1	2	3
3. Introduction to philosophy and concepts of nursing	1	2	3	4	5	0	1	2	3
4. Concepts of principles of teaching/ learning in nursing	1	2	3	4	5	0	1	2	3
5. Cultural diversity and implications for nursing	1	2	3	4	5	0	1	2	3
6. Community health nursing	1	2	3	4	5	0	1	2	3
7. Management of nursing care	1	2	3	4	5	0	1	2	3
8. Primary care nursing	1	2	3	4	5	0	1	2	3
9. Tertiary care nursing	1	2	3	4	5	0	1	2	3
10. Implications for drug therapy for nurses	1	2	3	4	5	0	1	2	3
11. Clinical practicum	1	2	3	4	5	0	1	2	3
12. Issues in nursing	1	2	3	4	5	0	1	2	3

VIII. How important were your educational experiences to increasing your concern and sensitivity to the following issues?

0 = Not Applicable
1 = Not Important
2 = Little Importance
3 = Somewhat Important
4 = Important
5 = Very Important

1. Concern with social issues   0 1 2 3 4 5
2. Concern with professional standards   0 1 2 3 4 5
3. Concern that patients are treated with   0 1 2 3 4 5
   dignity
4. Concerned with confidentiality of patient   0 1 2 3 4 5
   information
5. Concerned with patient rights   0 1 2 3 4 5
6. Concerned with fostering better rela-   0 1 2 3 4 5
   tionships with difficult and/or "undesir-
   able" patients
7. Concerned with the quality of care for   0 1 2 3 4 5
   incurably ill patients
8. Concerned with the unethical and/or   0 1 2 3 4 5
   incompetent conduct of colleagues

IX.   If you had it to do over again, would you still enroll in the nursing program?

___ 1. Yes
___ 2. No
___ 3. Don't know

X.   Please comment on the skills or areas of knowledge that should be added, strengthened, or eliminated.

XI.   Please add any additional comments or suggestions that you have about your nursing program.

Thank You For Your Cooperation!

Index

A

Accenting cue, 78
Acceptance rating, 237-238
Achievement, tests of, 66-67
Activities
  role playing, 96-99
  simulation gaming, 125-130
  value program, 57
Administrators, 226-228
Advisors, instructors as, 251-252
Affective domain, 2-3, 44
  assessment of training, 141-239
  communication skills in, 101, 103
  education of the, 3, 65, 71-140
  and interview skills, 196
  and simulation games, 110-116
  teaching objectives for, 48-60,
    207-217
  training handbook for, 130
Alcoholism, 22
Analysis. *See* Moral analysis
Anchor points, 170
Assessment
  See also Evaluation
  behavioral orientation to, 164-173
  checklist for self, 181-182
  of faculty advisory role, 251-252
  of faculty effectiveness, 245-251
  of former students, 254-269
  of instructional plans, 252-254

instruments for, 141-239
psychometric, 141-163
Attitudes
  changes in, 163
  continuum of, 156
  direction of, 148
  of instructors, 73
  and measurement limitations,
    162-164
  position of, 156-163
  preassessment of, 60-62
  psychometric assessment of,
    142-163
  and role playing, 95
  of students, 61-62
  and values, 11-15
  variables of, 157
Attending behavior, 101, 103,
  198-199
Attention, 52
Audience, learner as, 46
Audiovisual aids, 65-66
Awareness
  See also Empathy
  and receiving behavior, 51-52
  in students, 1-2

B

Behavior
  assessment of, 141-239

attending, 101, 103, 198-199
and attitude inconsistency, 162
developmental stages of, 4-10
and game rules, 113
of instructors, 73
measurement of, 42
and motivation, 63-65
nonverbal, 77-79, 198-199
observation of group, 229-235
orientation assessment of, 164-189
orienting of, 15
postassessment of, 66-67
professional, 11-12
repeating of, 15
research in, 11
and role playing, 107-108
sampling of, 169
setting objectives for, 44-60
value-laden, 3
written description of, 182-189
Behavior modification, 141-142
interview for, 202
Behavioral orientation assessment,
164-173
Behaviorally Anchored Rating
Scale, 171
Behaviorism, 141-142
Beliefs
and behavior, 13
and values, 56-57
Biases
of observer, 165
in student evaluations, 251

C

Care. See Patient care
Career patterns, 255
Case studies
anecdotal records, 54
Heinz's dilemma, 7
method of, 85-95
of nursing dilemmas, 118-124

and values inquiry, 19-22
Characterization, as learning
outcome, 50, 58-60
Checklists
for affective assessment, 176-182
for group observation, 229-235
for new administrators, 226-228
Choices, rank ordering of, 33-34
Clarification
of faculty expectations, 141-142
and questioning, 81
Classroom
achievement tests for, 207-217
psychological climate of, 76-77,
110-111
teaching strategies for, 71-140
Closure
instructional, 98-99
in role playing, 97-99
Code for Nurses, 11-12, 16-17, 24,
36-37
Cognitive domain, 44-46
Cognitive moral analysis. See Moral
development
Cognitive objectives, 66
Commitment. See Beliefs
Communication
in interviews, 198-202
skills of, 101, 103
Community building, 74
Complementing cue, 78
Conscience, development of, 7, 24
Consequences, and values, 12-14
Consensual location scaling, 156-163
Content, behavioral, 46
Context evaluation, 242
Construct, and attitudes, 143
Contradicting cue, 78
Costs/benefits evaluation, 243
Counseling, 142
and assessment, 189-207
Course evaluation, 245
Curriculum
and attitudes, 12
design of, 2-3, 41-68

and simulation games, 111
values clarification in, 17-19
Cues, 77-79

D

Data
  interpretation of, 206
  from interviews, 189
Decisions, value-laden, 15, 28
Design
  See also Planning
  of simulation games, 112-114
  systematic instructional, 41-68
Development. *See* Moral development
Dilemmas
  case studies of, 86, 118-124
  moral, 4, 10-11
  Nursing Dilemma Test, 11
Discriminal dispersion, 156
Discussion
  benefits of, 84
  in groups, 71-85
  in role playing, 98
Doctrines, ethical, 23
Documentation
  of behavior, 141-143
  of instructional programs, 241
Domains
  See also Affective domain
  of learning, 44-46

E

Education
  See also Teaching
  affective, 3-4, 71-140
  and moral development, 1-27
Educators
  See also Instructors
  nursing, 41-42
Empathy
  as affective skill, 197
  rating scale for, 236-239

Employer survey, 254, 258-261
Errors, in ratings, 173-174
Essay tests, 212-217
Ethics
  Kantian, 10-11, 23
  normative and applied, 2-3, 23-25
  principles of, 7
Evaluation
  See also Assessment; Rating scales
  of affective objectives, 207-217
  as component of meaning, 148
  by employers, 254, 258-261
  environment of, 169
  of essay questions, 213
  of input, 243
  of instruction, 241-257
  of instructional revision, 241
  of listening skills, 196
  of nursing demand, 255
  of planning, 252-254
  and postassessment, 66-67
  and preassessment, 60-62
  psychometric, 141-163
  of role playing, 99-100, 104
  by self, 181-182
  strategies of, 41-68
  by students, 246-251
  traditional, 207-217
Exercises
  See also Role playing; Simulation
    games
  for values clarification, 28-37
  for values inquiry, 38-39
Extention questions, 81

F

Facilitation
  See also Teaching
  facilitator's handbook, 130
  of learning, 114-115
  in role playing, 97-99
Faculty. *See* Instructors

Feedback
  in instruction, 42
  in interviews, 197
  rating of, 237-238
Feelings
  See also Affective domain
  empathy, 236-239
  reflecting of, 199-200

G

Games. *See* Simulation games
Goals
  education, 19
  of follow-up studies, 256
  of instruction, 42-48
  of nursing education, 67-68
  in simulation games, 113
Graduates, questionnaire for, 262-269
Grid, of values, 32
Groups, 71-85
  behavior in, 229-235
  Group Cognitive Map, The, 74-76
  handbook for facilitators, 130
  size and mix, 72

H

Halo effect, in scales, 173
Health science education. *See* Education
tion

I

Incidents, in case studies, 118-124
Instruction
  See also Teaching
  design and planning of, 41-68,
    112-114
  methods of, 71-140
  systems model for, 241
Instructional revision, 67-68, 241-257

Instructors
  as advisors, 251-252
  affective skills of, 196-198
  attitudes of, 73
  effectiveness measure of, 245-251
  rating of, 154-155
  and simulations, 112
  skills of, 96, 202
Instrumental-relativist orientation, 5
Instruments, rating, 246-251
Interpersonal concordance orienta-
    tion, 6
Interpretive questions, 90-91, 94
Interviews
  for assessment, 189-207
  and behavior modification, 202
  experiential, 194-196
  questionnaire for, 190-191

J

Johari window, 246-247
Judgment
  See also Decisions
  moral, 2-3

L

Law-and-order orientation, 6
Leadership, in groups, 78-79
Learning
  affective outcomes of, 49
  assessment of, 241
  by case study, 7, 19-22, 54, 85-95
  competency-based, 42
  domains of, 44
  in groups, 74-77
  preassessment of, 60-62
  by role playing, 96
  by simulation gaming, 9, 108-116
  strategies for, 62-65
  styles of, 64-65
  systematic approach to, 41-68

use of dilemmas for, 118-124
of values, 14
Legalistic orientation, 6
Likert scales, 141, 143-148, 221-225
Listening skills, 52, 196

M

Maintenance, as group function,
229-231
Meaning components, 148-156
Measurement
See also Evaluation
of affective behavior, 141-239
of student performance, 244-245
Media, instructional, 65-66
Meta ethics, 23
Methods
assessment of, 252-254
of instruction, 71-140
Model
of attitude position, 156
of evaluation, 257
of instructional systems, 41, 241
of problem-solving, 87, 93
of program evaluation, 242-244
of simulation games, 125-129
Moral analysis, 1-11
and ethics, 23
Moral development
See also Values
cognitive, 10-11, 25
and education, 1-11
theories of, 10, 25
and values inquiry, 19-23
Moral education. *See* Education
Motivation
of choices, 11-22
theory of, 63-65

N

Normative ethics, 23-26
Norms, professional, 24

Nurses
See also Students
Code for, 11-12, 36-37
educational goals for, 1-2, 67-68
ethics of, 24
evaluating demand for, 255
instruction of, 41-68
Nursing Board Examination Score,
243
Nursing Dilemma Test, 11
preparation for teaching, 254
self-assessment of, 181-182
values of, 16-17

O

Obedience/punishment orientation, 5
Objectives
affective, 2-3, 44-60
assessment of, 141-163
for discussion method, 72
of follow-up studies, 256
instructional, 42-48
and media aids, 65-66
preassessment, 60-62
and simulation games, 111
and teaching methods, 63
Observation
of behaviors, 164-189, 229-235
time of, 174
Operant conditioning. *See* Behavior
modification
Opinion statements, 159
Organization, as learning outcome,
50, 57-58
Orientation, in moral development,
5-11

P

Paraphrasing, 199
Patient care
satisfaction scale of, 221-225
and values, 12

Patterns, of values, 12-15
Performance measurement, 244-245
Philosophy
    of ethics, 23-26
    of moral development, 7, 10-11
Planning
    affective objectives, 48
    anecdotal records, 186-188
    for checklist use, 179-181
    evaluation of, 252-254
    group discussions, 72-73
    of instruction, 41-68
    for preassessment, 60-62
    role playing, 96
    simulation games, 110-114
Polarity, in scales, 148-156
Postassessment, 66-67
Post-graduate questionnaire, 262-269
Potency, as meaning component, 148
Practice, clinical, 254
Principles, ethical, 7
Problem-solving
    and case studies, 86
    games for, 112, 125-140
    joint, 201-202
    and value inquiry, 20-22
Process
    and attitude measures, 163
    evaluation, 243-246
    instructional, 241
Product evaluation, 243-244, 254-269
Professionals
    ethics of, 24
    and values, 16-17
Programs
    evaluation of, 242-244
    of value activities, 57-59
Projective techniques, 54
Prompting, 79
Psychometric assessment, 141-163
Psychomotor domain, 44
    media aids for, 66

Q

Questionnaires
    graduate follow-up, 262-269
    informational, 190-191
    of patient satisfaction, 221-225
    for student's employer, 258-261
Questions
    in case study method, 90-91
    models of, 79-84, 244

R

Rating
    See also Evaluation; Rating scales
    of communication skills, 101, 103
    of faculty, 246-251
    of listening skills, 52
    of students, 60-62
Rating scales
    for behavioral observation, 164-173
    forced choice, 167, 169
    graphic, 166
    interpretation of, 163
    Likert, 141, 143-148, 221-225
    numerical, 165
    ordered, 156-163
    position labeling, 152
    for psychometric assessment,
        141-163
    rank ordered, 167
    reliability and validity of, 173-176
    Semantic Differential, 141, 148-150
    Thurstone, 156-163
    of warmth, 172-173
Rationale, written, 43
Reasoning
    and ethics, 23-25
    moral, 4-10
Receiving, as learning outcome,
    49-52
Records, anecdotal, 182-189
Reinforcement
    and behavioral change, 141-142
    of responses, 82-84

Relating cues, 78
Reliability
  and anecdotal records, 188
  of attitude measures, 163
  of Likert-scaling, 147-148
  of Semantic Differential scales,
    155-156
  of Thurstone scales, 160-162
Repeating cue, 78
Reports, anecdotal records, 182-189
Research
  See also Reliability
  on interviews, 206-207
  in moral education, 10-11
  and scales, 147-148, 155-156
  in self-assessment, 181-182
  and simulation games, 110
  of student evaluations, 248-251
Responding, as learning outcome, 49,
  53-55
Responses
  and alternative test items, 208-210
  biases in, 162
  hostile, 205-206
Results
  of faculty evaluations, 249
  interpretation of scales, 163
  use of for change, 256-257
Risser Patient Satisfaction Scale,
  221-225
Role playing, 95-108
  directed, 104-107
  open-ended, 99-101
  structured, 102-104

S

Scales. *See* Rating scales
Scholarship, morality of, 1-2
Scoring
  of empathy scale, 239
  of essay tests, 214-217
  of Likert-type scale, 145
  semantic differential scales, 153

Selective perception, 184
Selective retention, 185
Self-assessment, and checklists,
  181-182
Semantic Differential Scales, 60-62,
  141, 148-156
Simulation
  case study method, 85-95
Simulation games, 108-116, 126-129,
  131-140
Skills
  affective, 48-60, 95, 196-197
  in discussions, 79-84
  listening, 196
  rating of communication, 101, 103
  in self-assessment, 181
Social contracts, 6
Stages
  of moral development, 4
Standards, of choice, 15
Strategies
  for affective training, 71-140
  for evaluation, 41-68
  for learning, 62-65
  preassessment, 60-62
  for value clarification, 17-19
Students
  awareness of, 1-21, 51-52
  employer survey of, 254, 258-261
  evaluation of faculty, 246-251
  follow-up studies of, 255-256,
    262-269
  and group discussion, 71-85
  mobility of, 255
  motivation of, 63-65
  performance measurement of,
    244-245
  preassessment of, 60-62
  response modalities of, 66
  and role playing, 95
  socialization of, 110
  stimulation of, 79-84
Substituting cue, 78
Systems
  models of planning, 42-43, 241
  of values, 13-14

T

Task functions, of groups, 232-233
Taxonomy, of affective objectives,
   48-60
Teaching
   See also Instruction
   by case study method, 85-95
   of ethics, 23-25
   evaluation of, 246-251
   media aids in, 65-66
   methods of, 62-65
   of nurses, 41
   objectives, 2-3
   preparation for, 254
   revision of, 67-68, 241-257
   by role playing, 95-108
   through simulations, 114
   strategies for, 71-140
   systems model for, 43
   using incidents, 19-22
   value-laden, 14
   of values clarification, 17-19
Terminology, of affective education, 3
Tests, 41
   essay items, 212-217
   multiple-choice, 210-212
   and postassessment, 66-67
   preassessment, 60
   supply-type items, 208-210
   and traditional evaluations, 207-217
Textbooks, 65·
   evaluation of, 253
Theories
   of behaviorism, 141-142
   of communication, 205
   of learning motivation, 63-65
   of moral and values education, 2-27

Thurstone scale, 141, 156-163
Training
   See also Instruction; Teaching
   in rating scale use, 169-172
Traits, and measurement errors,
   174-176

V

Validity
   of Likert scaling, 147-148
   of rating scale construction,
      173-176
   of Semantic Differential scales,
      155-156
   of Thurstone scales, 160-162
Values
   acceptance of, 55
   activities programs of, 57
   complex of, 58-59
   continuum of, 28-31
   indicators of, 32-33, 54
   introjection of, 12
   and judgments, 28
   nonmoral, 3
   patterns of, 16, 18
   preference for, 56
   psychometric assessment of, 141-163
      141-163
   system organization of, 57-58
   voting exercise, 35-36
Values clarification, 2
   exercises, 28-37
   theory of, 11-19
Values inquiry, 2, 19
   exercises, 38-39
Valuing
   as learning outcome, 49, 55-57
   process criteria, 13